Secrets of Wellness

staying healthy with natural hygiene

Secrets of Wellness

staying healthy with natural hygiene

ACHARYA S. SWAMINATHAN

First published 2005

ISBN 978-81-8328-436-3

Published by
Wisdom Tree
4779/23 Ansari Road,
Darya Ganj, New Delhi-110002
Ph.: 23247966/67/68
wisdomtreebooks@gmail.com

Printed in India

Dedicated to
Acharya Lakshmana Sarma

Contents

	Preface	*ix*
1.	Health Maxims	1
1.	Unity of Disease	16
2.	Unity of Health and Disease	22
3.	Unity of Food and Medicine	26
4.	Unity of Cause	31
5.	Unity of Treatment	36
6.	Law of Cause and Effect	43
7.	Principle of Non-violence	48
8.	Vital Economy	58
9.	What is *Prana*?	69
10.	Successful Piloting of One's Life	80
11.	Facing *Prarabdha* sans Misery	86
12.	Total Approach	96

Preface

Health is a positive state of well-being of the body and mind. It is not mere absence of a so-called disease condition.

Health must be deserved before one can desire it. In other words, one should by leading a well-ordered daily life and the care one devotes to keeping the body clean would qualify him for being called healthy.

The science of natural hygiene which deals with the subject of health in the most rational manner cannot be treated at par with health maintained through all kinds of medication. It is not an alternate system of medicine, though nowadays most people adopt this as a last resort to cure their disease condition, when all other systems fail. Though the disease gets radically cured, this does not mean that Nature cure is one which deals with healing of disease alone. Though the nomenclature Nature cure has stuck to it the world over, the ideal name for it should be natural hygiene, i.e. science of health based upon the laws of Nature governing human health and happiness. These laws are eternal, immutable and inviolable.

I was introduced to the subject in a very dramatic manner. A sudden transformation took place just in one day. It was the holy day of Sivaratri in February 1948 when Sri Swami Pranava Brahmendra Ananda Saraswati initiated me into the mysteries of this science. This person put me on to Acharya

Lakshmana Sarma for learning the laws, principles and theories of the science in depth. The latter, who was a fountain of knowledge, steeped in Advaitic philosophy transmitted the message of Mother Nature to me.

That this science of natural hygiene has a philosophy of its own is to be thoroughly understood by every health-seeker. Once the philosophy is understood, a person would not care to look around for remedies from any other source. Health can be had only through healthy means and not through any remedies whatsoever.

Remedies are galore the world over for relieving the symptoms of various disease conditions. These may afford apparent relief. For some time a person may be free from symptoms and he may mistake that he has been cured of that disease. But he cannot even retain his health, not to talk of improving his health. Natural hygiene alone guides man on how he can retain his health and progressively improve his level of health further and further. As for those who are having subnormal health are 'said to be suffering' from this or that disease condition. Natural hygiene here again clearly guides as to how he can regain his health the only sane and safe way.

The author is convinced that without a clear understanding of the theories, principles and laws that form the basis of natural hygiene, a follower may not be able to benefit very much. Hence the author has described the theories, principles and laws in this book. These have to be studied in depth by every health-seeker. The enlightenment that he will get by a thorough knowledge of these principles would give him the greatest reward.

The healing power is within every person, that is, the real doctor. Give that healing power the much-needed opportunity to assert itself and set the condition inside right.

In days of modern civilisation no one can be said to be ideally healthy. Hence everyone, including the person who is now free from the disease condition, has to become a follower of natural hygiene. In other words, natural hygiene is the science by following which the ill can become well, the well can become better and the better can become still better. This science is to be learnt and practised by all. Each follower can become totally self-reliant.

There is no substitute for the basic knowledge of health presented here. Health is your birthright and you can have it throughout your life. Disease is not inevitable.

The author owes this knowledge to Sri Swami Pranava Brahmendra Ananda Saraswati, Parmahamsa Swami Sivananda Saraswati and Acharya Lakshmana Sarma. May the blessings of these gurus fall upon all readers.

Acharya Swaminathan

health maxims
(positive indicators of health)

What is health?

- The human being is a triple unity of body, mind and spirit. Health involves caring for the body, caring for the mind and caring for the spirit as Nature intends the human being to take care of them.
- Health is a positive state of well-being of the body, the mind and intellect (not just the absence of disease); the health level of a person is assessed by finding out the extent to which the indicators of health are present in him.
- In the state of health there is an evenness in the distribution of heat (known as body temperature) all over the body.
- A healthy person experiences a unique sense of lightness—not to be mistaken for weakness in the body, enabling him to carry on the external and internal activities easily.
- In a state of health there is a feeling of comfort (*sukham*) all the time with this feeling arising out of the body's internal cleanliness.
- Hunger is an indication of health; the keenness for hunger in a state of health enables the person to enjoy the taste of natural food. Good digestion is an additional bonus.

- A healthy person should experience the state of deep sleep for a few hours at night daily. On getting up from the bed next morning, he experiences a feeling of freshness and energy.
- The bloodstream inside is clean and the skeletal and muscular systems are in tone. A healthy person discharges his daily duties very comfortably and without any aversion to work.
- All his eliminatory organs, without being overtaxed will discharge their functions satisfactorily ensuring freedom from toxaemia from within.

Basic Nature cure or natural hygiene is that branch of science of life which deals with the care of the organism in a state of disease. It recognises law of health, which is also the law of cure and by obedience to this law, health and healing are both obtained. It includes all hygienic measures such as proper dieting, fasting, rest and relaxation, exercise (active, corrective and recreational), *pranayama*, sunbathing and hydrotherapy, which form part of the five-fold food medicine. There is no place in this science for drugs of any kind or for electrical, mechanical or other applications or so-called aids, which ultimately impair or endanger health. Non-violence to the human organism is accepted as the basic principle governing the application of all Nature cure measures advocated herein.

Life power (*prana shakti*)

- What activates every cell and every tissue within the body is the life power which is super physical, super chemical, incapable of being manufactured or obtained either from within or from outside through any activity.

- This life power is endowed on the infant at birth by Mother Nature. In other words, it is inherent in the organism.
- The life power so endowed in the newborn is kept as a reserve within and is known as *prana shakti*. As to where the reserve is kept is unknown to man.
- To enable the body, the mind, etc. to carry on their internal and external functions, day after day, a small quantum of power is released from the reserve. Such release takes place when one is asleep at night.
- The energy that is made available to the person on rising up from bed can be termed as the vital power or *jeevan shakti*.
- There can be no action—physical or mental, external or internal—without a corresponding expenditure of power. The power so spent on any activity, be it big or small, is that of *jeevan shakti*.
- In a body that is clean inside, the activities that go on within the body are termed as physiological activities. In a body that has become unclean, the activity of *jeevan shakti* (elimination of toxic matter from within) is called pathological activity.
- There is no dividing line as it were between physiological and pathological activities. In reality it is one continuous biological activity that goes on inside.
- The symptoms do not signify disease. Suppressing the symptoms through the use of drugs is illogical, irrational and unhygienic.
- At the back of all diseases lies a cause which no drugs can reach.
- Due to the adoption of unhygienic habits of life, quite an

amount of *jeevan shakti* gets wasted day after day, the eliminatory activities of the body suffer adversely and the body becomes unclean internally.

- Adoption of unhygienic activities results in enervation. Enervation leads to defective elimination, which in turn results in accumulation of un-eliminated toxic matter (a state known as toxaemia). Toxaemia is the universal basic cause of disease, be it the common cold, the dreaded cancer or AIDS.
- *Jeevan shakti* prevents storage of dirty matter within the body. When some matter accumulates over a period of time, *jeevan shakti* suspends, as it were, most of the functions of the body and concentrates on eliminating the accumulated dirty matter, with the person experiencing symptoms like the common cold, cough, boils, loose motions, vomiting, etc. This occurs in the acute stage of the disease.
- The disease is called acute because *jeeven shakti* is very vigorous (or acute) in this period. The term acute is not to be mistaken for 'serious'.
- The passive cause of disease is the accumulation of dirty matter within, while the active cause, therefore, is the *jeevan shakti*.
- Vigorous elimination of unwanted foreign matter from within lasts only for a short time. As a large part of the available *jeevan shakti* is engaged in elimination, the person concerned experiences weakness in his skeleton muscles, lack of hunger, coated tongue and inability to attend to simple intellectual activities.
- Such an acute form of disease is in reality intended to help the person to restore his internal sanitation back to normalcy.

- When the symptoms of acute disease are sought to be suppressed through the use of drugs or in any other mechanical manner without employing any drugs, the internal uncleanliness of the body goes on increasing slowly and steadily, leading to the onset of one or the other type of chronic disease.
- Unlike acute disease which lasts only for two to four days at a time, chronic disease, e.g. asthma, bronchitis, high blood pressure, low blood pressure, heart trouble, joint diseases, sluggish liver, etc. can manifest themselves for all the twelve months of the year. In this state the daily availability of *jeevan shakti* gets lowered and the toxic matter inside steadily increases. Use of drugs and continued adoption of unhygienic living habits only worsen the health level within.
- When the basic cause of chronic disease is not understood by the sufferer and when the symptoms are sought to be allayed by the use of drug or any other mechanical manner, disregarding the working of the law of cause and effect, the person concerned hops on to the third stage of disease termed as destructive disease, e.g. epilepsy, tuberculosis, cancer, AIDS, etc.
- A disease in its primary stage is termed as acute; in its state of 'graduation', it turns chronic and the 'post-graduate' state of disease manifests as a destructive disease. Hence wisdom lies in not allowing the progression of the disease to occur in the body.

Prevention of disease

- All destructive diseases can be effectively prevented—and this is the only sane method of prevention—by not 'treating' chronic disease through drugs or any other mechanical manner. Similarly all chronic diseases can be prevented by not 'treating' acute disease irrationally through drugs, etc.

- As the state of disease implies some discomfort, minor or major, to the sufferer, the wise should know not only to prevent chronic and destructive diseases but also practically apply such knowledge in day-to-day life. This is what the science of natural hygiene elaborates in great detail.
- Any attempt to 'prevent' any state of disease through so-called inoculations and vaccinations, etc. is but a futile effort, for only living hygienically can prevent disease. *Health is the way; there is no way to health.*
- Whenever a person takes a drug, a vaccination or an inoculation, etc., he is only transplanting the disease for future use.
- Let not the acute disease be suppressed. No chronic disease can develop in the person. The question of developing a destructive disease will not arise.
- When a patient suffering from a chronic or destructive disease takes to a hygienic way of living and proceeds to rebuild his health the sane and safe way, the vital power or *jeevan shakti* in him becomes a part of the internal cleansing process, bringing on from time to time the healing crisis (for a short period) for the specific purpose of raising the patient's health level.

Unity

- All disease signifies tissue uncleanliness within though the cause of all disease is one. There are not so many diseases. There is only one disease, i.e. lowered level of health. This principle is termed as the 'unity of disease'.

- Disease can be radically cured by restoration of the health level of the patient through adoption of a hygienic way of living. The cause of all disease being one, the treatment is also one, namely, restoration of health level back to normal by living in tune with the laws of health. This is known as 'unity of treatment'.
- When there is but only a minor accumulation of toxaemia within and when *jeevan shakti* occasionally (say once in six or eight months) initiates a vigorous activity to eliminate it, such elimination takes place for improving the health of the body. This principle is known as the 'unity of health and disease'.
- Even during the chronic and destructive stages of a disease when natural hygiene is followed, life's 'will to health' asserts itself periodically through cleansing the body by bringing on the healing crises.
- The principle of unity of the cause elucidates that the cause of all disease is one.
- The common notion prevalent in the society is that a diseased person has to take in some medicine to cure his disease. The science of natural hygiene calls upon man to avoid the use of poisons (which all drugs are) and take to a sensible and limited intake of natural food during the disease stage for radically curing the disease. This principle is termed as 'unity of food and medicine'.
- What food is healthy and what food can help build up the health level of a person can alone serve as a medicine when a person falls ill. What is not food in health can never be medicine in a disease state.

The five-fold food

- The human body is made up of five elements of Nature, viz. *akash* (loosely translated as 'ether'), air, natural light (*agni*), water and earth (meaning thereby the edible plant foods grown in soil).
- Each of these five elements constitutes food for man. Any deficiency in the supply of any of these elements will result in an internal imbalance or ill health. As the principle of unity of food and medicine operates all through, only these five elements can serve as man's medicine. This principle is known as 'five-fold food medicine'.
- Chemicals, metallic products and every kind of poison taken out from the bodies of animals, reptiles, etc. can neither be food nor medicine for man.
- As Dr Henry Lindlahr has effectively put it: "If all the *materia medica* as at present known were to be sunk to the bottom of the sea, it will be all the better for mankind and all the worse for the fishes."
- In place of *materia medica* that is seen in different systems of medication, natural hygiene advocates *materia hygienica* as a positive aid to health. Poisons and non-food products can never serve the purpose of nectar. Let Nature be the guide and let her dictates be followed scrupulously.

The germ theory of disease

- Some micro-organisms (germs, bacilli, microbes, etc.) may be seen in pathogenic matter inside but to mistake germs as being responsible for disease is totally wrong.
- In many disease conditions, germ activity may be present but killing the necessary germs through drugs, etc. may

give some temporary symptomatic relief to the patient. But the fact remains that the health level never improves. It goes on steadily worsening in every germ-hunter.

- Natural hygiene clearly proves that germs are not the cause of disease. If the germ theory were true, no disease can be cured through adoption of natural hygiene. The fact is that even medical failures are radically cured only through the adoption of natural hygiene.
- If the germ theory were true there can be no disease without the so-called causative germs clearly visible inside. The fact is that in so many disease conditions, the so-called causative germs are not at all seen when the disease is in its early stages.
- The germ is but a cleaner, a scavenger recruited by Mother Nature for clearing the dirt from within. As noted playwright, George Bernard Shaw, has put it: "These human beings suffering from horrible diseases infect us who are microbes and you doctors pretend that it is we who infect them." It is plainly admitted even by bacteriologists that the so-called medicines administered for killing the germs really add to the resistance power of the germs. The germs subjected to such torture become drug resistant. A stage is reached when no drug whatever can ever 'control' the symptoms of the disease.
- Let not suppression of symptoms through drugs be adopted.
- Chronic and destructive diseases will be totally out of the picture. Kill not the scavenger who has come in at the behest of Mother Nature to cleanse the body from within.

Food and energy

- The prevalent notion mistakenly considered as scientific that food is the source of energy is the reason why numerous persons eat without being hungry. They eat even when they clearly know that they cannot digest the food taken in by them.
- The intake of food by a person may create a psychological feeling that 'he has supplied energy to the body', which makes him temporarily feel better even though no physiological benefit is ultimately derived by the eater.
- What activates every cell and tissue within the organism is the *jeevan shakti,* which cannot be produced by the food taken inside the body. Digestion of food is a vital action necessitating the expenditure of *jeevan shakti* (vital power). It is unscientific to hold that an activity, which involves expenditure of power, supplies power to the body.
- As Acharya Lakshmana Sarma, the eminent health authority, has practically proved that food is a tax on vitality, common sense decrees that there should be the minimum of tax imposed on vitality, i.e. just to the extent needed and no more.
- Where the food eaten is natural and where it is digested properly the body gets therefrom the requisite blood sugar, amino acids, the needed fatty acids, the different types of vitamins and mineral salts, the necessary enzymes, trace elements, water and the cellulose or roughage required for keeping the body chemistry in order. All these are just 'matter' and not energy.
- When the requisite vitamins, etc. are supplied to the body, the body is able to keep the structure of the different organs in proper shape. In that ideal condition *jeevan shakti*

can manifest itself through the different organs very easily, i.e. with the least expenditure of *jeevan shakti*. Where the wrong type of food is supplied and where many of these materials are not available inside the body, the concerned structures become weak and that is why weakness is felt by the person concerned. Thus food is not a source of energy; it is a medium through which energy is expressed.

Healthy dietetics

- Eat only when hungry and that too moderately (i.e. not more than half the stomach load at any given time and not more than twice a day). The load on the digestive system becomes unbearable if a person eats three or four times a day.
- Work and digestion do not go together. When there is work, keep the stomach as light as possible. At this stage take only raw vegetables, seasonal fruits or juices.
- The main meal should be taken at the end of the day when all work is over. This way one can go to sleep comfortably without the world disturbing him. Even the night meal has to be moderate in quantity.
- Keep away from all bottled foods, tinned foods, manufactured and preserved foods, etc. Take only natural foods, that is foods as given to human kind by Nature.
- Refining of cereals, etc. robs the foodgrains of many nutrients like vitamins, minerals, etc.; Sir William Arbuthnot Lane has put it aptly: "The whiter the bread the sooner you are dead."
- Whatever can be consumed raw, uncooked, let that be taken raw. Whatever needs cooking, let it be steamed. Let

it be cooked through the steam cooker. Over-cooking should be avoided.

- Fruits ripened artificially through chemicals or in cold storage are unfit for human health. Milk, to serve the purpose of milk, should be fresh. The longer the milk is kept on the shelves the more useless it becomes. Pasteurised milk is stale milk.
- Where good, fresh milk is not available, man must remind himself that none other than human beings consume the milk of other animals. It is possible to live healthy without milk and milk products. Tens and thousands of vegetarians (who have nothing to do with any of the animal products) are living even today in different parts of the globe. If the vegetarian diet is properly planned, one can live without milk or milk products.
- The body requires a moderate supply of predominantly alkaline foods day after day. Such foods are vegetables, fruits, etc. which should predominate in the diet, and can be supplemented by a small quantity of unrefined cereals, etc.
- Predominantly acidic foods such as refined cereals, de-husked pulses and grams, refined flour, white sugar, stale milk, flesh foods, eggs, confectionery and hydrogenated oils have a deleterious impact on human health.

Vital economy and non-violence

- As *jeevan shakti* is wasted when one adopts unhygienic activities, common sense decrees that only hygienic habits be adopted in daily life. These have to be adopted in tune with the principle of vital economy and non-violence to produce the best results.

- The principle of vital economy, a principle which finds mention only in the science of natural hygiene, states that only such actions are to be performed by the human being that entail the least possible expenditure of *jeevan shakti*.
- Sticking to the principle of non-violence in daily life ensures the correct observance of the principles of vital economy.
- Periodical fasting even when one is healthy ensures the observance of vital economy.
- The daily programme of living has to be so designed that no organ in the body is over-worked, that no organ is (through the use of drugs or mechanical, electrical or other contrivances) forced to function in a particular manner, that basic needs of living are supplied in the right and balanced proportion as it is essential to see that no violence whatever is inflicted on any organ inside. Every act of violence enervates the organism and the health-seeker has to acquire the requisite knowledge on what results and what does not result in such violence.
- Fast of a short duration of one or two days may be observed even when one is healthy.
- In acute diseases total fasting would help in radically curing the disease quickly. In chronic diseases, partial fasting is to be resorted to by the concerned patient. In destructive diseases, approach to fasting is to be resorted and when conditions improve positively, partial fasting may be undertaken.
- Fasting is not starvation. The fear that fasting can weaken the person is baseless.
- As and when there are healing crises, treat them on par with acute disease and fast accordingly.

- Every health-promoting application like non-violent *pranayama*, the spinal bath, the non-violent enema, etc. have to be resorted to well within the limits imposed by the principles of vital economy and non-violence. If this is borne in mind, ideal results will ensue.
- Attempting to get symptomatic relief from distressing symptoms through the use of mechanical or electrical contrivances may involve drugless methods but as the relief, even if obtained through these contrivances, is in violation of the law of cause and effect, these methods/ applications should not find a place in the programme of one who has taken to natural hygiene. Natural hygiene has enough practical guidance to give to the sufferer to enable him to achieve the needed symptomatic relief. Let these be done sensibly and non-violently.
- A calm mind hastens recovery from disease. A calm mind ensures that the glands and nerves in the organism work far better.
- The very adoption of a disciplined way of life advocated by natural hygiene helps in controlling the mind as also in controlling the sense organs properly.
- The discipline involved here will calm down the mind, improving the power of intellect considerably.
- Such adoption of natural hygiene in daily life combined with daily prayers to the Almighty and proper attention devoted to the cultivation of virtues like humility, sincerity, magnanimity, etc. would go a long way in enabling the human being to live and move on the path towards perfection.
- What is needed is understanding and sincere application of the principles involved.

Adoption of total approach

While every hygienic habit is by itself welcome, it is unwise to choose one such habit alone, swear by it and follow it to the exclusion of various other hygienic habits. It would be completely futile. Let the total approach be adopted by every health-seeker.

unity of disease

Same cause

Natural hygiene holds that all disease—whatever nomenclature it may assume in different persons or in the same person at different times—is due to the accumulation of foreign matter (so called because what constitutes that matter is foreign to the body). This foreign matter is the cause of all diseases. Natural hygiene holds that all disease is one at its root. This is signified by the principle of 'unity of disease'.

The hygienic stand is rather baffling to the common man who gullibly swallows what is doled out to him by the drug or dope-dispenser. Thus he fails to understand the scientific basis behind the principle of unity of disease. He asks how could angina pectoris or coronary sclerosis be the same as the common cold, sinusitis, etc.

Here is the explanation. Medicos also admit that without some pathogenic matter in some part of the body there cannot be a disease. The existence of this pathogenic matter in any part of the body is sought to be located by diagnostic methods. Having found the 'obnoxious substance' within, the medicos proceed to analyse it and find the existence of micro-organisms in that substance—like pneumococcus, the gonococcus, etc., which is, according to them, 'the mischief maker' in the formation of that pathogenic matter. In quite some cases the so-called 'mischievous' micro-organism cannot even be spotted, by the analysts. But even there they insist that some bacillus or virus, etc. must be present!

Is the micro-organism the cause for the formation of pathogenic matter or is it a product of the pathogenic matter? Some micro-organism or the other is found in all types of pathogenic matter and it is futile to deny the existence of that organism. Instead of simply declaring that the micro-organism is the sole cause of the disease condition in the patient, natural hygienists plead that the real cause of disease be probed into not through blind acceptance of the 'germ theory of disease' but by practical observation (on humans) of how the disease is radically cured.

It is an admitted fact that many incurable diseases get radically cured within a reasonable time if the patient follows the principles of natural hygiene. Having agreed to follow natural hygiene, the patient keeps away from all drugs. He does not attempt to 'exterminate' the so-called 'offenders' from within. He simply takes to diet reform and improves his digestion/assimilative capacity slowly and steadily. He breathes better. He takes air-baths and sunbaths. He fasts occasionally but very cheerfully. He totally disregards the 'offensive germs' and without making any attempt to kill them, he recovers totally.

If the germ theory had been correct and scientific, can this be a practical proposition? The bare fact is that hundreds of cases defying medical treatment are cured within the four walls of one's home. If the germ theory of disease has a scientific basis behind it, then natural hygiene ought to be a dismal failure in every case. That natural hygiene does not fail the follower is known to every dispassionate observer.

Cause of disease

The proof of the pudding is in its eating. The successful results that follow and the practical applications of the principles of natural hygiene are proof enough that the so-called offensive micro-organisms in the pathogenic matter are not the cause for the existence of that matter inside the body. Practical observation reveals that the existence of pathogenic matter in the body is but a development due to defective elimination. Through natural hygiene, the body is helped to heal itself by observance of 'vital economy'—a principle rarely recognised and which involves elimination of the pathogenic matter through the normal eliminatory (or occasionally even in an extraordinary manner) channels. Once that offensive matter has been eliminated through the practical application of the principles of natural hygiene, the disease can no more be there. The cure is effected and that too is a radical cure for one who follows natural hygiene goes on progressively improving his health level.

That the pathogenic matter found in 'various types of disease' happens to be different from one another and is located in different parts of the human body is an admitted fact. This fact by itself cannot establish that every disease is different from every other disease condition.

That the human organism is not just a community of different organs set out in a particular form but is a single integrated whole regulated by the life power, *prana shakti,* within has to be realised by every health-seeker. Defective elimination does result in the accumulation of foreign matter. The real cause of disease is that which has brought about defective elimination. There are ever so many enervating habits in modern man, many of them even 'foisted' on him by various circumstances and the social environment.

- Wrong posture in sitting, sleeping, walking and while at work.
- Lack of requisite physical activity in the form of exercise.
- Ill-fitting footwear.
- Wearing tight dresses or dresses made of synthetic fibre.
- Living and/or working in ill-ventilated places.
- Sluggish breathing.
- Eating without hunger.
- Consuming denatured, devitaminsed, demineralised foods and 'drinks', often containing insecticides, pesticides and other chemicals in them.
- Working on loaded stomach.
- Drinking water without thirst.
- Addiction to stimulants, tea, coffee, cola drinks, etc.
- Falling prey to smoking and drinking habit.
- Harbouring the wrong notion that drugs alone can cure diseases, by regularly consuming one drug or the other.
- Not having the right attitude to life and its problems.
- Subjecting oneself to tension all the time, mistaking 'livelihood' to be synonymous with life.
- Exposing oneself to the effect of radiation through X-rays, television, etc.

The above list is illustrative and not exhaustive. Anyone can easily deduce what the other enervants can be. Each of these enervating habits is a tax on a person's vitality. And the person who chooses to live in the conventional way chartered out for him by vested interests has, at any time, very little vitality left in him to keep his body internally clean. What leads to defective elimination—by the skin, by the lungs, by the kidneys and by the bowels—is hinted above. The style of life usually adopted by most modern men and women is the real cause of disease.

Unhygienic living

As the cause is one (which could be covered by the term 'unhygienic living') and as the patent types of disease are like the leaves of a tree fed by a single root and trunk, natural hygiene holds that all disease is one.

Life power or *prana shakti* is endowed by Mother Nature on the infant at birth. It is kept, as it were, hidden from the understanding of man as a vital reserve within. All this cannot be taken out at one time and utilised by man. The minimum energy required for carrying on the day's activities is released by the vital reserve. When a person is asleep, it is this limited energy (known as *jeevan shakti*) that enables the individual to live day after day. This point is elaborately explained in the chapter on 'Vital Economy'.

Unity in diversity

All mankind is one though there are so many human kinds, each looking different from the other. The 'principle of unity' pervades all over the universe. He alone is wise who can perceive the unity behind the apparent diversity. One who cannot perceive this truth is bound to be misled, though he might go to the extent of claiming himself to be a well-cultured man. His mind may well be deluding him and under the effect of such delusion (termed as *maya* in Indian philosophy), he might turn a deaf ear to those whom he considers to be opposed to his way of thinking. Once a person is so deluded, he shuts himself off from all understanding. He is literally installed in an ivory tower. This unfortunately happens to be the case with most people who claim to be authorities on science.

The scientist too, whether he likes it or not, has to see the 'unity in diversity'. If science deals with the diversities without recognising the unity behind them, science may even be called atheistic.

Whether one likes it or not, science has come to occupy the central role in modern civilisation. What is called scientific temper is very good to adopt as it signifies impartiality and search for truth. If only the scientists were to understand the subtle truth behind Vedic culture, if only they were prepared to apply the universal truth enshrined in Vedic culture to their scientific approach and interpretation, the world would be the ultimate gainer.

Here then is the secret of the principle of 'unity of disease'. Those that fail to understand the facts are likely to be hopping from disease to disease, till death 'delivers' them from all problems. Let every health-seeker delve deep into the truth and discover for himself that natural hygiene is a way of life and not just a therapy to be adopted at times and to be given up at other times.

unity of health and disease

Having understood that diseases are fundamentally one, that the basic cause of all diseases is one as explained in the previous chapter, let us now proceed to comprehend matters relating to health and disease in detail.

Health and disease are inter-related

It is commonly thought the world over that disease is an entity having its own existence. It is also believed that the disease process is set in by some forces (microbe, virus, bacillus, germ and what not) inimical to health and that if the disease is not 'properly treated' the health level of the concerned individual gets seriously impaired. In many cases, description of the situation in this regard by the mass media–newspapers, journals, radio, television, etc.—is so frightening that people are terrified out of their wits. The fright gets more aggravated when the same patient is 'diagnosed' by different doctors in various ways. Where physicians and surgeons vary in diagnosing the same patient, it is the poor patient who becomes the victim! The science of natural hygiene, on the other hand, helps the layman to understand the facts of the case as they are. It is quite possible that the symptoms experienced by the patient may be troublesome, but the moment he understands the real situation within his body, his worries will be considerably lessened and he will learn how to face his problems.

As Acharya Lakshmana Sarma say: *Disease is in reality a diminution in the level of health and cure lies in the restoration of health by living hygienically* (in the most comprehensive sense of the term).

An ordinary individual in the modern society gets rather confused when told that disease has no existence of its own. He says: "When there are so many specific diseases in modern society, especially the communicable and contagious ones, how can one say that disease has no existence?"

Latent and patent stages of disease

Disease can arise only in an unhealthy and unclean body. Logically the unclean body has some toxic matter inside it—some may call it pathogenic matter—which is responsible for the onset of disease. In some cases the matter gets eliminated either slowly or vigorously, and in other cases, it is retained without being eliminated. When elimination is slow the symptoms experienced by the patient include discomfort. Such a disease process is called 'patent disease'. Where the pathogenic matter is inside the body without any specific eliminatory process the patient has the disease in its latent stage, though the discomfort is not so intense at this stage.

Of these two stages of disease—the latent and patent, which is to be preferred for getting back to normal health? A little reflection will indicate that the patent one is better because in this case the eliminative process is on and if not interfered with, the patient's health level improves as it is relieved of the dirt from within slowly, steadily.

All activities inside the body are initiated and carried on by the vital power within. Even this patent disease has been initiated by the very vital power ostensibly for cleaning the body from within. The vital power within is always working health-ward and the patent disease process is a vital effort towards re-establishment of health. It is life's expression of its 'will to health'. Wisdom decrees that such an eliminative process should not be interfered with in any way.

Sane way to health

While wrong, unhygienic living leads to accumulation of foreign matter within, the vital power's vigorous effort in eliminating the foreign matter for restoring internal sanitation within (which at normal times keeps everything in order by carrying on all physiological activities in a systematic manner) continues unabated. Discretion lies in recognising the truth behind this statement.

And this is what we Nature-curists mean by the term 'unity of health and disease'. Let not the disease process be mistaken or misinterpreted as a process initiated by forces inimical to the life of man. It is a process initiated by the 'vital power' within. So, set right the condition inside the body to normalise all its functions once again.

It is wrong and illogical to say that the physiological and pathological processes are opposed to each other. There is no dividing line between the physiological process and pathological process; in reality, it is one continuous biological activity.

Considering the pathological process as a serious threat to health, let no attempt be made to take in drugs (miscalled as medicines) for symptomatic relief day in and day out.

The modern world is replete with instances where persons keep taking drugs and suffering all the time from 'some' disease or the other. Experience of Nature-curists the world over proves that radical cure of the disease (let the nomenclature appended to disease be anything) can be resorted to when the biological process inside is allowed without any hindrance to restore the sanitation in the body through sane and sensible hygienic living. Let the disease process be initiated by the 'vital power' to re-establish health in its fullest sense of the term.

Cure lies in the restoration of health and not in suppressing the symptoms of disease. When the disease in its earlier stages termed as being in acute stage is suppressed through symptomatic treatment, the patient hops on to the chronic stage of disease, wherein he suffers throughout the year. And when the suppressive treatment is resorted to in the chronic stage for some months or longer, then the patient hops on to the destructive stage of the disease with very little vitality left in him to enable the body to become clean once again.

Drug way is not the way to health. It is the grand royal road to more and more disease. Disease can be eradicated only through hygienic living. In the acute stage, the disease should actually be welcomed and allowed to go its own way for the purpose of re-establishing health.

unity of food and medicine

Proper intake of food

One of the basic needs of living is food, the others being air, water, sunshine, exercise, rest, etc. Food comprises of items from the plant kingdom to enable living beings to derive the nutrients intended to keep the cells and tissues in good working order. Every healthy individual experiences hunger twice a day. This sensation within him indicates that his digestive organs are ready to receive and act upon the food consumed by the person.

Foods produced by the plant kingdom and consumed fairly fresh by the individual in moderate doses and keeping in mind the other dietetic rules of discipline, can be digested without difficulty. During digestion, the nutrients released, like blood sugar, proteins (amino acids), some fatty acids, the various vitamins and mineral salts, trace elements, etc. are utilised by us for carrying out various activities. The roughage in the natural food helps the alimentary canal to move the food from one end to the other, especially in the bowel. It helps to move the faecal matter in time so that the person is free from constipation.

Thus, the food sensibly taken by a healthy individual is intended to maintain his health level and improve it step by step.

Three stages of disease

As stated in the preceding chapters the disease condition occurring in an individual is fundamentally due to a fall in his health level brought about by unhygienic living. If the fall in the health level is not much and if there is an adequate quantum of *jeevan shakti* within, the person experiences acute disease (for two or three days) once in six, eight or twelve months. If the fall in the health level is more and consequently the quantum of *jeevan shakti* within drops, the person passes through the second stage of disease known as chronic disease. This lasts all through one's life (unless the individual is wise enough to adopt natural hygiene to reverse the gear and progress towards improvement of health). If stage of chronic disease is 'treated' through drugs the patient hops on to the third stage of disease, called the destructive disease (cancer, tuberculosis, etc.). Even in such a destructive stage of disease where the *jeevan shakti* within is at a very low level, Mother Nature is ready to help, provided natural hygiene is adopted in tune with the laws of life.

The treatment prescribed under natural hygiene for patients is given according to the following stages— in the acute stage; in the chronic stage; and in the destructive stage of disease to enable the affected body to be cleansed internally before its restoration to health.

In all systems of medication there is a 'specific medicine' for each disease condition. But Nature cure is the only treatment devoid of drugs. What could be the medicines for patients undergoing Nature cure treatment?

The substance given to the patient ostensibly to help him recover his health is termed 'medicine' and every system of medication claims that the substances in each *materia medica* is a medicine. Now what does this word 'medicine' connote? Why is it that in Nature cure we do not approve of these so-called medicines? Why is it that in Nature cure a drugless treatment is prescribed?

The word 'medicine' is derived from the Latin root *medicina,* a substance the consumption of which promotes the health of the patient. Can any of these substances now normally used as medicines be deemed as 'health-promoting'? The answer is 'no' in every case because the medicines are prescribed with the sole purpose of keeping the symptoms of disease 'under control', offering the patient some symptomatic relief for a time. In fact, it is admitted that many of these medicines have side-effects and after-effects, which are far worse than the original disease condition sought to be cured by medicines. It may be noted that there is a group of diseases known as 'iatrogenic diseases', which mean 'drug-caused diseases.'

Can such substances heal the patient in the real sense of the term? In our view these cannot, and hence in Nature cure we assert that the disease can be cured only through food which promotes the real health of the patient. Hence, we hold that what is food in health and what as food can improve the health of a healthy person can alone serve as medicine for the sick and this is what is communicated through the principle of the 'unity of food and medicine'.

Hinder not the healing process

The healing power within the patient wants that healing activities should not be hindered in any manner. If such a hindrance is removed, the healing will be automatic. Let me, at this stage, list out in what manner the modern man hinders the healing process and makes health recovery almost impossible.

- He takes in drugs—the so-called medicines—with the sole intention of suppressing the symptoms and attaining symptomatic relief by hook or by crook.

- He takes in food at both times of the day on the assumption that food is a source of energy. He goes to the extent of questioning as to how he can get along with his daily normal activities without consuming his 'normal' food at least twice a day.
- The person takes in his usual stimulants like tea, coffee, etc.
- He continues to live a tense life without caring to find out how a tension-free life is led.

As stated earlier, in a state of health, food is a substance which sustains life and enables the eater to maintain his blood purity and blood circulation.

In a condition of disease, the digestion process slackens down—sometimes it remains absent for a few days. If this principle is fully grasped by the patient and if he is convinced that the food taken beyond his actual needs would surely hinder the healing process, if he further understands that the vital nutrients in positive foods alone can help his system to regain normalcy before long, he would gladly take 'this medicine' to the total exclusion of the poisonous drugs.

Yes, 'food is our medicine' according to the principles of natural hygiene. Food alone can be the proper medicine. Now, the food to be taken by the patient has to be determined according to his condition. If the disease is in acute form, there will be no hunger and the patient is advised to take only tender coconut water or some juice, thrice or four times a day in strictly moderate doses. This condition will not last for more than three or four days at a time.

If it is a case of chronic disease then the patient would take some time to recover. In the sub-acute state of chronic disease, i.e. the symptoms of chronic disease would not be outwardly severe, the person can take tender coconut water or some raw juice, once in the morning (8 a.m.) and again late in the afternoon (at 4 or 4.30 p.m.). At mid-day he may take a plate of raw vegetables and at night he can take some seasonal fruit. When the symptoms are outwardly very severe and seem very uncomfortable, and the patient is advised to follow the programme prescribed earlier for the acute stage of the disease and gradually the health level will improve.

When the patient is in the destructive stage his hunger level dips. He is advised to live on tender coconut water or juice taken four times a day. He cannot digest more than this at this stage.

As the condition improves, his health level will improve. He can then adopt the programme advised for chronics earlier. He can improve his health level slowly and steadily.

Proper regulation in the quantity of food consumed and proper attention to the quality of food are the two vital points to be borne in mind.

Patients even in chronic and destructive stages of disease can slowly and steadily rebuild their health. Their digestion level will slowly and steadily improve. This dietetic programme will ensure ample rest to their nervous and glandular systems by observing the principle of 'vital economy'.

Let the patient understand the principles involved and follow the programme cheerfully and hopefully, without any fear or doubt in his mind. What is taken by the patient is medicinal food which removes all hindrances to the healing process and supplies all the needed nutrients like vitamins, mineral salts, etc. to the physical organism.

What is food in health can also be medicine in disease. What is not food in health—drugs, synthetic vitamins, synthetic minerals, processed foods, etc.,—can never serve the purpose of medicine.

unity of cause

It is the life power or *prana shakti* inherent in the human organism that carries on the physiological activities. It is this very power that ensures that no unwanted matter gets accumulated in the organism. In a state of health, the bowels, the kidneys, the skin and the lungs are engaged in eliminating the unwanted matter without causing discomfort to the human organism. The matter to be eliminated is not much and such elimination takes place easily with the least expenditure of 'vital power'. So the patient feels lighter after elimination without getting exhausted. The only elimination that goes on is through the lungs, but as the lungs are not congested and are in tone with the rest of the body, elimination through this channel proceeds smoothly.

Accumulation of toxic matter

When the human being indulges in unhygienic living and as a consequence wastes his 'vital power', the eliminatory organs are unable to work satisfactorily. As a result, 'foreign matter' gets accumulated inside the body. This accumulation is due to the fact that the matter to be eliminated (faeces, urea, uric acid and other waste products, or improper elimination of carbon dioxide through the lungs, or the skin, cell and tissue, etc.) is more than what can conveniently be eliminated. It is because such energy is wasted elsewhere in the body that the person feels enervated. This accumulated toxaemia becomes the passive cause of disease, be it common cold or the dreaded disease called cancer.

For every action taking place in the world there is a passive (material) and an active (efficient) cause. For instance, when an earthen pot is being made, the clay is the material cause and the potter, the efficient cause. Similarly for disease too there is a material cause and an efficient cause. In common parlance, the symptoms represent the disease. As the symptoms vary from one condition to another, it is commonly mistaken that a man has many diseases. What is meant by the term 'unity of disease' is unity of the cause of disease. What is commonly known as disease is only an effect and the cause of disease is within the organism. The cause—toxaemia—is after all only the presence of foreign matter.

How can toxaemia, an inert substance, cause disease? Readers may note that I have described toxaemia as the passive cause of disease. The active cause of disease is the 'vital power' or *jeevan shakti*.

Toxaemia is accumulation of waste within, which has to be eliminated by the body. Without such elimination taking place, the body cannot become clean internally, that is, health cannot be regained. But in this state, matter to be eliminated is excessive, elimination of which needs extra impetus. And so the 'vital power' works vigorously to induce elimination and this is what disease is.

For further classification of the readers, when the daily eliminatory organs cannot eliminate the faecal matter, urinary wastes, etc., the body becomes internally insanitary day by day. When such internal insanitation builds up progressively, the body becomes more and more unclean internally. It is at this stage that the 'vital power' begins its extraordinary activity of vigorously eliminating the accumulated dirty matter from within.

Latent and patent phases

So long as the dirty matter is within, the patient feels uneasy; he is internally having disease. This is the latent phase of disease. This internal discomfort felt by the concerned person is not recognised as disease. Apparently it is not patent outside; it is not diagnosable. When on a particular day, the 'vital power' within diverts its attention to clearing this toxic matter, acute symptoms are felt. The disease becomes patent.

In this patent state, the disease manifests in the form of common cold, cough, loose motions, boils, fever, etc. This active effort of 'vital power' in eliminating the foreign matter from inside is called the body's pathological activity. It is assumed that as there are acute and uncomfortable symptoms while this pathological activity is going on, the pathological activity is 'opposed' to the physiological activities. As the symptoms are somewhat relieved due to suppression of these pathological activities, it is claimed that the patient is better and the disease is under control.

This is a completely wrong. Acharya Lakshmana Sarma in his magnum opus *Swadheena Swasthya Mahavidya* says:

"The activity of the prana shakti *in a human body which is fairly clean within is termed physiological activity. The activity of the* prana shakti *inside the body, which is very much unclean, is called pathological activity. In other words, the pathological activity is also initiated by the life power within. Let it be noted that when there is no life power in the body, when the body is dead, there can no more disease within. There can be no purposive activity in a body having no life within it."*

When the toxaemic matter inside the body is in excess, when the available life power within is at a fairly high level, then vital power puts in vigorous effort to eliminate the dirty matter for restoring the health of the person. The disease process becomes acute or vigorous.

If such an acute process is not suppressed through violent drugs, the disease inside the human body cannot progress towards the chronic or destructive stage. If modern humanity is witnessing chronic and destructive diseases, it is due to the drug suppression of acute diseases. Those who follow natural hygiene in their daily life will never suffer from any chronic or destructive disease.

In chronic and destructive diseases also the cause is the presence of toxaemic matter within which through drug treatment has not been allowed to be eliminated. The cause of all diseases is the same. This principle is known as the 'unity of cause'.

What is *prana?*

Life power is super physical as well as super chemical. It is not the product of any activity within the organism or from outside. It is inherent in the organism and difficult to comprehend. An ordinary man cannot understand but persons steeped in spirituality, can understand what this life power is.

What has been termed as 'life power' is designated as *prana shakti* in Sanskrit and practically in all Indian languages. *Prana* is the total quantum of the power given to the individual at birth. It is 'stored' inside the person and every day when the person is asleep, a small quantity of this power is taken out of the vital reserve and made available to him on getting up from bed, for carrying out the internal and external activities during the next day. What is thus made available for the day's activity could be termed as 'vital power'.

The fact that only the spiritually advanced can comprehend what life power is does not mean that the average man/woman in the world cannot practise natural hygiene and benefit therefrom. The science of natural hygiene is so simple that everyone can understand and practise the art of healthful living.

In the world outside too there is unity. Behind the apparent diversity that presents itself before our eyes we have to observe the underlying unity. In other words, to the common man life is a 'mystery' and will continue to be so. The *Kathopanishad* (2.1.10) boldly declares: *"He, who is incapable of seeing the unity behind the diversity, should continue to suffer all along."* The science of natural hygiene deals with recovery in health and promotion of health as its main objects. Natural hygiene or Nature cure unequivocally declares that all disease is fundamentally one—that there is an underlying unity between health and disease, that what is food for the healthy can alone be medicine for the sick and further, the mode of treatment to be adopted for the radical cure of disease should also be one.

unity of treatment

In modern times even providing symptomatic relief to patients is claimed to be a successful method of treatment and any remedy which suppresses the symptoms instantly is hailed as a breakthrough, showing that the person resorting to it lacks something in his health and that he wants to instantly make up for the deficiency.

For the purpose of restoring the internal body condition back to normalcy, he wants to hit at a health recovery plan, which he can adopt. In other words, the person who wants to be treated should know his problem and whatever method of treatment he adopts must be logical, that is, in tune with the law of cause and effect. The treatment must be one which has convinced him that it is the rational method to be adopted.

It may be argued that many health problems are so highly 'technical' that an ordinary person can never understand them, let alone plan for a treatment of them by himself. Most practitioners of the different systems of medicine happen to exploit this human weakness as the common man is not familiar with the real facts. So long as this feeling of helplessness in the vast majority of the people (as compared to the total population of the world, the number of 'practitioners' is but a very small percentage of the population and the 'patients' constitute a very large majority) persists, the problem of disease will continue to be present. Incidences of a few diseases may have dropped but the number of patients (suffering from different kinds of diseases) keeps on increasing. 'Treatment facilities' may go on increasing but the 'helplessness' in the people continues without any reduction. The number of patients will never go down and, as a result, no improvement is seen in the average health level of the people as a whole.

Science and technology are coming up with new and newer inventions. It is said that in this era of information explosion, where anyone in the world can just press a button and get the required information instantly, there are many diseases which are incurable and which man has to suffer all through his life. Is it not time for the entire humanity to delve deep into the problems of disease causation and treatment, casting aside all prevalent theories and temporary solutions?

A number of people in the modern world have cast aside the prevalent theories and charted out a new path for themselves. They have recovered from their so-called incurable diseases radically through what is commonly termed as Nature cure approach. This is based on an understanding of Nature's unalterable laws governing human health and happiness.

Treatment of disease

How should disease be treated? Does not the word 'treatment' imply total health recovery, making it unnecessary for the patient to continue taking his 'medicine' all through life?

Every prevalent system of medication 'accepts' that the healing power is inside man. All that the different systems say is that they are helping the healing power in man from outside. While this is what is claimed by every system of medication, it is seen that the *materia medica* of each of these systems is constantly undergoing changes. The 'wonder drugs' of, say the 1960s have turned to be 'blunder drugs' of 1990s and new wonder drugs have taken their place to turn into 'blunder' drugs in 30 years again. This has been going on during the past two or three centuries or more. Would not a clear analysis of the situation reveal that what was claimed to be helpful for mankind has not really delivered the goods?

Every patient wants to be cured as quickly as possible. This is but human nature. When a person has a disease, he experiences a certain amount of discomfort in his body—the symptoms of the disease—and he wishes to be relieved of that internal discomfort at the earliest possible.

Suppose a person has an unbearable 'burning sensation' in his stomach whenever his stomach is empty, let him be relieved of his burning sensation, provided the remedy he applies for achieving his objective does not cause him further complications inside the body in future. This is why in Nature cure we object to patients resorting to symptomatic treatment.

There are various systems of medication, each viewing 'each disease condition as separate from every other' and holding that each disease condition needs a specific medicine in a specified dose a specified number of times in a day. In other words, each system of medication recognises the existence of disease as an entity and that 'it should be fought within through a specific medicine'.

Every system is of the view that each 'medicine' helps the patient in curing his disease. In other words, healing is effected through this or that medicine prescribed by the system of medicine. It is not as if every patient feels better after medication; in many cases, it has to be accepted that the disease is incurable and 'in order to keep disease under control', the medicine(s) must be continued indefinitely. Where even 'one disease' is said to have been cured within a few months, the person gets 'another disease', that is, there are repeated episodes of various diseases periodically.

Healing is Nature's sole prerogative. It is the life power that heals the body. For any system of medication to claim that healing is effected by its medicines is totally illogical and incorrect.

Five unities

In the previous chapters entitled unity of disease, unity of health and disease, unity of food and medicine and unity of cause, the rationale behind the Nature cure approach has been explained logically, rationally and scientifically. If what has been presented is recognised as the real cause of disease, if the truth that the medicine used for treatment should not be a poison (non-food product) with serious side-effects and after-effects later is accepted, then the problem of treatment would be very much nearer to a solution.

Let the five theories concerning 'unities' be understood thoroughly. Your faith in Nature cure will be strengthened and you will not waver.

No one can change or alter Nature's laws. Man has essentially to submit himself to those laws; he has no alternative left for him. If man is to be free from chronic and destructive diseases he has to humbly submit to Mother Nature and rectify his/her past mistakes in living.

Now let us try to understand how to get healed through Nature. As this vital theory of unity of treatment happens to elude most modern minds, so more elaboration on the subject is set out here.

As has been made clear, there is only one disease—the cause of it being one; hence the treatment is also one, namely to restore health back to normalcy through obedience to Nature's laws. That is the 'unity of treatment'.

A diseased person wants to be healed. How can he heal himself? He can heal himself only by improving his health level, for, it is the diminution in his health level that has led to his disease. In other words, there can be no treatment of disease without restoring the health level.

Acharya Lakshmana Sarma has aptly said: "*Disease is in reality but a diminution in the level of health; cure (or treatment) lies in the recovery of health by living according to laws of Nature.*"

We, of the Nature cure school, would prefer to adopt the *materia hygienica* in place of *materia medica* which goes on changing decade by decade. Let the treatment of the patient be done through this *materia hygienica* which involves intake of Nature's edible (non-poisonous) *satvik* herbs, vegetables, fruits, etc. This has been clarified in the earlier chapter on 'Unity of Food and Medicine'.

How can the health level be improved? This can be achieved only by ensuring that all habits of living, physical and mental, are based upon sound theories and principles. He has to give up his earlier unhygienic habits of living and start caring for his body, caring for his mind and caring for the spirit as Nature intends him to care for them. This and this alone can be the rational method for health recovery.

Even if one is not suffering from any type of disease, his health level may not be ideal, or digestion is not up to the mark, or sleep is not so refreshing, or even minor problems are a common daily feature creating tension.

To whichever category you belong, there is a common rational health-building plan, which anyone can adopt. In fact, I would like to even keep away from using the word treatment and employ the constructive term 'rebuild health'. *How can health be rebuilt?*

It can be done by reforming one's style of life in such a manner that all the physiological activities begin to improve day by day. Thus, the internal sanitation brought about by better working of the eliminatory organs is normalised. The nervous and glandular systems are also given their due share of rest. The mode of breathing is not only improved but also moved towards near perfection by doing rhythmic breathing exercises so that more oxygen is made available to every cell and tissue. A rational plan is devised to enable man to go through his daily job free from tension.

Therefore, the healing plan of the treatment suggested by the science of Nature cure is more or less the same for all patients.

Nature cure teaches what food to eat, how much to eat to meet the basic needs of living and to regulate life, take the non-violent enema, the cooling abdominal wet pack, the spinal bath, the sunbath, external help like massage to the ailing body, and do some bodily exercise to ensure better blood circulation.

In preparing a treatment plan for a patient, we bear all these points in mind. Nature cure does not 'treat' diseases; it helps patients to build up their health. Even fairly healthy individuals can add to their health in the same manner.

The above is the 'treatment plan' that we recommend to everyone who wants to restore his health back to normalcy. The science of Nature cure has no remedies; it tells patients, "remove the basic cause of disease by adopting right living". Normally before a patient takes to any 'treatment', he submits himself to clinical tests in order to diagnose his disease. The results of such clinical tests may at best throw light on the state of affairs that is there at that time. Based upon 'these findings', one might even name or diagnose the disease. The question is, does the problem (root cause) get solved? Has any light been shed on what has been causing the regular fall in his health level?

In Nature cure, however, we study the case history of the patient from as far back a period as possible, study his style of living, that is, his habits, and correlate one with the other. We explain to the patient as to which of his unhygienic habits are responsible for the regular fall in his health level. We tell him how he can help himself by reforming his lifestyle as per Nature's unalterable laws.

Here lies the difference between the 'treatment' prescribed in other systems and the treatment plan adopted in Nature cure.

The various systems of medication now prevalent in the world mistake the symptoms of the disease and declare symptomatic relief as a cure. The fact is that none of the remedies used as medicine by these systems improves the health of man. No doubt in most cases symptomatic relief is experienced by the patients. But is that alone enough?

This is where the science of Nature cure administers a warning to all mankind. Whatever is suggested by the science of Nature cure is hygienic or health promoting. I am not referring only to foods or drinks but even to hygienic factors and influences, that have their impact on the improvement of human health.

law of cause and effect

The statement *'as you sow, so shall you reap'* forms the basis of the law of cause and effect. Unlike the man-made law, which can be amended, re-amended and even repealed, Nature's laws are eternal, immutable and inviolable.

In all fields of science man has necessarily to understand Nature's laws and follow them strictly; let it be the field of physics, chemistry or any other physical science. If so much 'progress' has been made through scientific research, it is just because the scientist is very careful in following the relevant laws.

Man had studied the law of gravity in great depth and he is able to fly heavy machines—aeroplanes, etc. up in the air just by ensuring that the conditions due to earth's gravity would not bring down the planes. Space research had become possible only because man's understanding of the relevant laws and practical application thereof are maintained very strictly.

But the scientist's over-confidence and over-assertion that he can ensure normalcy even while observing abnormal or subnormal ways of living has landed society in a dangerous situation. No one can either flout Nature's laws with impunity nor can he think of challenging them.

While in all other fields of science, the scientist and the inventors have to operate through lifeless machines and gadgets, in the field of health, the 'machine' through which man has to work and live in this world is not man-made. What distinguishes the living body (and the subtle power of the mind) from the lifeless machines and gadgets is that the very development of the body straight from the stage of conception on to mature adulthood is something which takes place automatically as designed by Nature.

It is the life power which makes the human body maintain the symbiosis in the various organs, regulate the organisation within and direct all its activities towards set purposes (at times disease, at times recovery and the like).

Let me at this stage make it very clear that I am neither opposed to the scientific approach nor to the adoption of the scientific temper. If science adopts the real scientific temper all through, there ought to be no difficulty whatsoever. What is denoted by the term 'scientific temper' is the scientist's readiness to go deep and logically into every problem facing him, bearing in mind the relevant laws of Nature which govern his field of research. I am only pleading with everyone to visualise, recognise and live in accordance with Nature's laws that govern human health and happiness. Of all these laws, the law of cause and effect is perhaps the most fundamental one. This law is inexorable—let not this fact be erased from the mind.

Internal sanitation

Hygiene is the science that deals with and explains the health of the body and mind. Hygiene implies cleanliness—not mere external cleanliness or sanitation but far more important than that—internal cleanliness or internal sanitation. Internal sanitation can be maintained at a near ideal level by man

- by ensuring that blood chemistry is normal—the blood containing all its constituents in proper proportion;

- by maintaining proper blood circulation all through his body. The twin objectives referred to above can be had only through proper and balanced supply of all the basic needs of living— *akash*, air, water, sunlight, food, activity, mental poise, etc.;
- by ensuring that he does not wastefully spend his life power within him;
- by keeping his nerves in tone (first by not upsetting the tone through improper nutrition and secondly, by practising the art of dealing with all problems/issues with a serene mind).

Life power within

I have to point out here that none of the physical sciences cares to dwell on questions like what life power is, how it operates in the human body, how it is wastefully spent and how it can be conserved for man's ultimate benefit. Not having even a vague idea of what life power is, modern medical science deals with the human body as if it were a machine made up of many spare parts and working mechanically. This is the reason why chronic and destructive diseases are on the increase the world over.

A patient of high blood pressure uses hypotensive (blood pressure reducing) drugs to bring down the pressure forcibly. Maybe for a few hours the patient looks normal, but has he become normal? Has his internal condition been normalised? Have the causative conditions of high blood pressure been set right radically? No. The drug is incapable of it. Unhygienic living, in the most comprehensive sense of the term, had led to the development of high blood pressure in the patient and only the adoption of hygienic living by him can set it right.

What has been stated above in regard to high blood

pressure can be applied *ipso facto* to every disease condition. Almost every therapy like electrical and mechanical contrivances, magneto-therapy, acupuncture, accupressure, reflexo-therapy, chromotherapy, urine therapy, the so-called *pranic* healing, etc. prevalent in the modern world deal with the body only mechanically, disregarding the life power within, disregarding the law of cause and effect.

The fact is that surgery too is disregarding the laws. The surgeon removes only the effect but cannot remove the cause. The cause left unattended can only worsen the latent condition of the patient (these worsened conditions being generally termed as post surgical complications, occurring commonly).

Here is a plea made to drug therapists who talk of the effectiveness of acupuncture, magneto-therapy, auto-urine therapy, etc.—reiterating their claim that these are able to give immediate relief to the sufferers. But do they not ignore the law of cause and effect? Affording immediate relief to the patient is claimed as curing the disease. Does this not amount to deceiving oneself? It is here that the interpretation of the law of dual effects makes the position very clear to the seeker.

Law of dual effects

The effectiveness of a particular method of treatment is to be judged not solely by the immediate effect brought into being by the 'treatment', but its ultimate effect on the human body. Most people seem to take notice of the immediate effect ignoring the ultimate one. Taking advantage of this human weakness, stimulants are advertised to be energisers, sedatives to be having the capacity to soothe the nervous system. What is the ultimate effect of each of such methods?

Tobacco does not calm down the nerves, does not steady the nerves but turns the user increasingly unsteady later. Coffee and tea do not energise the individual; they enervate him. Laxatives and purgatives do not cure constipation but confirm constipation. Insulin and insulin substitutes do not help the diabetic but confirm his diabetic condition forever. Let these truths sink into the mind of every sane individual and let him recognise that the ultimate effect is most important.

Basic Nature cure as expounded very lucidly by Acharya Lakshmana Sarma could be the sole saviour of mankind. Those that adopt Nature cure must keep away from mechanical, electrical or other contrivances mistakenly presented as natural methods.

Nature cure alone recognises the law of cause and effect as clarified by the law of dual effect. Just because this science of Nature cure is presented in the layman's language, let it not be misconstrued as unscientific.

In interpreting the law of cause and effect in any particular case, the term 'effect' should relate only to the ultimate effect and not to the immediate effect as the latter is non-existent since it is purely transitional, lasting but for a little while. The ultimate effect is the lasting effect and hence this alone can be 'the effect'.

Perhaps, the best explanation of the law of cause and effect has been given by Acharya Lakshmana Sarma, who says in his magnum opus *Swadheen Swasthya Mahavidya*: *"Almost every action of man has two effects: the immediate and the ultimate. The latter is opposed to the former. The former, i.e. the immediate effect is purely temporary (symptomatic). It is the ultimate effect of the action that is real; the former is not. Hence, let man's actions be chosen rightly. This is the logical step of a discerning person."*

principle of non-violence

What is meant by the term 'violence'? Every organ in the body can function efficiently and effectively only when work is given according to the internal needs bearing in mind the 'needs' of the body as a whole. The term 'normal work' implies that no organ is to be overworked in any way and that it should not be given any unusual work.

When a poison (miscalled medicine), which is not the basic need of the body, is forced into the body and when some organs inside the body are compelled to counteract, neutralise and eliminate that poison, it is an unusual work. When food is taken by an already overworked yet weak stomach, this too is an abnormal or unusual work. The vitality or *jeevan shakti* expended on normal activity cannot be called a waste of power. But any expenditure of vitality on an abnormal or unhygienic activity is logically a waste of power. Such wasteful activities imposed on any organ of the body constitute violence.

Conversely, power spent on normal hygienic activities strictly meant to satisfy the normal physiological needs of the body amounts to non-violence.

Health through non-violence

Acharya Lakshmana Sarma once said: *"If all the organs of the modern man were to meet in a round table conference, each of them will start revealing its tale of woes, explaining how it is being abused and how it is overworked. And all the organs would ultimately pass a 'motion of no confidence' against the man on the ground that he does not know how to manage his organs."* Different types of diseases of different organs of the body are fundamentally due to the violence imposed on the organs by the person concerned. Every insensible and unhygienic activity is violence.

Hence, every health-seeker should clearly know the relationship between non-violence and health and thus manage his daily programme so as not to impose any violence on any organ of his body or mind.

Every step/method that qualifies as non-violent in the light of the detailed explanations given in this chapter will also be in tune with the principle of 'vital economy'. In other words, what is violent will be in violation of the principle of vital economy.

While the truth has been elucidated in the earlier paragraphs, health-seekers may want an elaborate explanation of the terms violence and non-violence in relation to the different systems in the body and hence, I am furnishing here the relevant data to guide them along the right lines.

Digestive system

- **Violence:** Eating food when one is not hungry, or when one is tired or exhausted, or emotionally upset or when he is expected to do fairly heavy manual/mental work immediately after a meal.

  Non-violence: Eating only when one is hungry and fairly relaxed, when one is mentally calm and free from tension, when one can afford to take rest for an hour or two.

- **Violence:** Eating hurriedly, eating beyond one's digestive capacity or eating more than two times a day.

Non-violence: Taking care to chew each morsel of food thoroughly, eating moderately or rather frugally and eating but only two times a day (once around midday and next at the early part of night).

- **Violence:** Consuming denatured, devitalised, refined, packed, tinned, bottled and processed foods (as none of these is a 'natural' food).

  Non-violence: Taking in food produced by Mother Nature as whole and as fresh as practicable.

- **Violence:** Consuming fried food with condiments, spices, etc.

  Non-violence: Realising that each natural food has its own taste and odour, consuming each natural food sensibly, where possible raw or steamed, with as little condiments and spices as possible.

- **Violence:** Taking in food with very little of vegetables in them.

  Non-violence: Realising that vegetarianism is a vital factor in the building up of health, taking plenty of vegetables — raw and steamed in every meal.

- **Violence:** Consuming unseasonal vegetables (this applies also to fruits) taken out of cold storage.

  Non-violence: Taking in only vegetables/fruits which are seasonal and fresh.

- **Violence:** Consuming fruits artificially ripened through chemicals or fruits, which are sprayed with insecticides and pesticides (this also applies to vegetables).

  Non-violence: Consuming fruits ripened naturally in a fresh state. Fruits/vegetables with poison sprayed over them (which are carcinogenic) are unfit for human use.

- **Violence:** Drinking water during the meal and immediately after the meal.

  Non-violence: Taking in of water (strictly according to the sensation of thirst) approximately an hour before the meal, taking care not to drink water during the meal. If there is overpowering thirst after the meal, let small sips of water be taken just to satisfy the thirst glands in the tongue.

- **Violence:** Denying rest to the digestive system, taking in the scheduled meals day after day, even when one is ill.

  Non-violence: Undertaking a fast as and when needed for short periods to give the much-needed rest to the digestive system.

- **Violence:** Trying to 'overcome' constipation by straining oneself at stools or sitting too long on the pot or using purgatives and laxatives or enema.

  Non-violence: Practice of hygienic habits to tone up the bowels and using the non-violent enema as and when necessary.

Respiratory system

- **Violence:** Getting accustomed to sluggish breathing.

  Non-violence: Taking care to keep the lungs in tone by practising the non-violent *pranayama*.

- **Violence:** Always sitting in wrong posture or sleeping on a soft bed.

  Non-violence: Taking care to maintain the body posture in all conditions in the proper manner and sleeping only on a hard bed (with, of course, a clean bed sheet).

- **Violence:** Exposure to air pollution.

Non-violence: Ensuring that one's house and workplace are free of air pollution as far as possible.

- **Violence:** Under the wrong impression of 'strengthening' his lungs indulging in violent types of *pranayama* like *bhastrika, kapalbhati, sheetli, sheetkari,* etc.

  Non-violence: Realising that strength of the respiratory system cannot be forced on but that it could be had only by adoption of right living, doing the non-violent type of *pranayama* and avoiding the violent types (which are unsuitable for adoption by the tense man of modern times).

- **Violence:** Wearing tight clothes or exerting undue pressure over the system, thereby obstructing proper blood flow and supply of nerve energy (incidentally tight clothes over any part of the body are harmful).

  Non-violence: Wearing clothes which are slightly loose (leaving a column of air all the time in between one's skin and clothing).

- **Violence:** Wearing apparel made of synthetic yarn.

  Non-violence: Wearing only cotton clothes and just to the extent required, during winter wearing woollen clothes over the cotton ones.

Skeletal and muscular systems

- **Violence:** Lack of physical activity.

  Non-violence: Where the so-called normal life has no scope for physical activity, taking resort to light exercise to the extent needed to ensure that all organs of the body are benefited through it (just as over-eating is bad, similarly over-exercising is equally bad).

- **Violence:** Getting addicted to wrong postures while sitting, standing, working, etc.

  Non-violence: Taking proper and sensible care to maintain one's posture in the manner designed by Nature.

- **Violence:** Use of tight footwear (exerting a cramping effect on the feet) or use of high-heeled shoes or tight socks gripping the legs.

  Non-violence: Use of footwear made of leather (not plastic or any other synthetic material) as to provide enough comfort to the legs.

- **Violence:** Indulgence in dancing which exerts tremendous force on the tissues and bones of the thighs, legs and feet, resulting in development of flat foot and various other disease conditions of the lower limbs.

  Non-violence: Dancing to the extent needed (where it is one's profession or hobby) gracefully and non-violently moving the legs and tips of fingers of the hands as seen in classical dances like Bharatanatyam or losing oneself in the spirit of the dance) and avoiding exertion of any type on any muscle/tissue or bone in the leg region.

- **Violence:** Indulgence in so-called muscle building or 'height-increasing' exercises.

  Non-violence: Realising that the health of the muscular system is solely dependent upon hygienic living, let exercise be done well within one's limit and never beyond it. (It is worth remembering that too much of unwanted muscular tissue in the body is more of a burden on the heart.)

Nervous and glandular systems

- **Violence:** Indulging in any unhygienic activity especially over a period of time.

  Non-violence: Taking care to plan one's activities in tune with natural hygiene.

- **Violence:** Addiction to stimulants, narcotics, sedatives or drugs.

  Non-violence: Taking positive steps to keep every system in proper working order and keeping away from stimulants, sedatives etc.

- **Violence:** Addiction to smoking and alcohol.

  Non-violence: Strict adoption of temperance is necessary, bearing in mind that such adoption is hygienic and ethical.

- **Violence:** Exposing oneself to jarring sounds or indulging in wrestling, etc.

  Non-violence: Taking positive steps to ensure peace and solitude to the extent possible and resorting to constructive hobbies.

- **Violence:** Wearing clothes of synthetic yarn and ill-fitting footwear.

  Non-violence: Let clothing be for comfort and health. Clothes should be made of cotton and of wool, where necessary. Footwear should not be of plastic or of any stuff made of chemicals. Footwear should be such as to allow free movement of the legs even when worn. But the ideal situation would be to remove the footwear as and when one can do without it. Socks/stockings worn over the legs, inside the shoes should also be of cotton and not synthetic yarn, like nylon.

- **Violence:** Indulgence in outbursts of anger, rage or weeping; indulgence in emotional attitudes like envy, jealousy, greed, etc.; getting into mental states like worry, anxiety, melancholy, self-pity, depression and the like.

  Non-violence: As the subject covered is vast, it could briefly be stated here that the health-seeker will have to pay attention to the mind culture as elaborated by natural hygiene.

- **Violence:** Developing a fancy for sex literature, sexology, etc. Not to talk of physical indulgence alone, even mental indulgence in such topics will shock the nervous system of both man/woman.

  Non-violence: Realising that the ideal of total absence from sex is unattainable for most people in the world, develop a sane and safe attitude towards sex. Let it be realised that there are ever so many sensible ways of keeping oneself happy. Let actual sexual indulgence be limited. Self-restraint could be practised by almost everyone, if one desires.

Every action indulged in by a person in violation of law of cause and effect or law of dual effects would entail wasteful expenditure of vitality and hence every such action is deemed to be an act of violence. Conversely, every action that is in tune with the two laws referred to would not entail wasteful expenditure of vitality. The expenditure involved in such action could be deemed as 'sensible' only when such action is necessary in the interest of life and/or livelihood, when it is an unavoidable necessity.

Links with vital economy

The said principle of non-violence is very closely allied to the principle of vital economy, the observance of which is very essential for maintenance and improvement of health and in case of patients, for recovery of health.

Vital economy is that orderly way of life as ordained by the law of cause and effect and law of dual effects with the avowed object of maintaining order at the bodily as well as mental levels.

Vital economy implies that the person so channelises his vital energy or *jeevan shakti* as to ensure that all his basic needs of life are supplied in a balanced manner all the time.

If at all a person makes a slip here or there in his orderly way of life, there ought to be an instant awareness of the lapse by the person concerned. He repents, not superficially, not through words, but through his subsequent action, which later sets right the lapse with the least possible delay. In matters pertaining to livelihood, a person who observes the principle of vital economy is consequently able to execute his worldly duties by channelising his vital power positively without allowing any portion thereof to go waste.

What sustains a nation all through, even during times of crises, is the soundness of its economy. Similarly, what sustains a human body both in health and disease is the observance of vital economy in letter and spirit.

Let life be lived in such a manner as to enable a person to live long in a healthy condition and with a sense of fulfillment at the mental level. That is why the science of natural hygiene expects man to do more and guides him to live life on the principle of non-violence as elaborated in the preceding pages.

Vital economy implies a total realisation of the truth that the one and only power behind all physical and mental activities is the 'vital power' and that the health of a human being depends on proper utilisation of this power and avoidance of waste of this power on activities or actions which are unhygienic in nature.

What has been stated in this chapter has been derived from the knowledge given to the writer by his guru, Acharya Lakshmana Sarma who has elucidated the principles of non-violence and of vital economy for the benefit of mankind. Wisdom lies in observing the much-needed discipline in life so that one's future is healthy, happy and holy.

vital economy

Order and the Ordainer

There is an order behind the working of the human body and this order is wonderfully maintained all through life by a power — the power within. Even when a person is ill, the power within tries to restore the order by taking steps to clear the body of the accumulated dross (foreign matter). The same order is present in human beings in the entire world and indicates that there is an Ordainer who maintains this order in every case.

The life power within each living body is the power that matters. There is no power apart from this. No third person or machinery in the world can give energy or power to the other's body. Even the digestion of food, oxidation of food, the secretion of various digestive juices, the absorption of food in the bloodstream are functions of the life power. Hence, the health-seeker who likes to maintain his health should have a clear understanding of what life power is, what is its origin, how it is expended and how at a particular time it gets exhausted in the body, leading to his death.

As life power is not a product of any activity in the world and as it is not 'manufactured' out of something else, a mystery surrounds it. However, it is obvious to every discerning person that life power is inherent in every living organism, in every cell of the living organism. As every cell, every tissue and every organ discharges its work, the power gets spent. But there is no way to replenish the power that has been spent. So the mystery turns a little more curious.

Life power is not something which can be taken out of the body, which can be measured, or subjected to so-called scientific scrutiny. When at the point of death, life departs from the body, everyone around including the technocrat or the scientist has to keep silent.

In Sanskrit, as also in other Indian languages, the life power is called *prana shakti.* It is *prana* that is behind the working of the lungs all twenty-four hours of the day, making him breathe in and breathe out rhythmically. It is *prana* that is behind the systole and diastole of the heart and thus the circulatory system. It is *prana* that is behind the working of the digestive system, the absorption of food and the elimination of the faecal matter and urine. It is *prana* that is behind the working of the senses—eyes, the ears, the skin, the nose and the tongue.

The truth is that *prana* is present in every living cell. It is *prana* that gives the somatic awareness to each cell by which the latter knows what is to be assimilated and what is to be eliminated. It is *prana* that maintains the symbiosis among the different systems of the body so essential for maintenance of health.

This is not an earthly power produced by someone on earth in some mechanical manner. It is a divine gift. Every human being is endowed with *prana* at the time of birth. The person concerned is expected to live perhaps for eighty or ninety years but all the power cannot be expanded in one day. Day by day it is released from within to carry on the day's activity from some secret vital reserve. As to where that vital reserve is located continues to be the greatest secret. That *prana* in each living body is limited in quantity and that it owes its origin to the Creator, is only implied, as it cannot be proved.

The Ordainer in each particular case seems to be *prana*. But the source of all *prana* is the Supreme Being; so that the Supreme Being is the Ordainer.

Vital reserve

A person is expected to live for a number of years and that much *prana* is present in his organism to enable him to live that long. That is the vital reserve or the reserve of *prana shakti*.

But what is needed for a day's expenditure for carrying out different actions, different functions of the different organs/tissues/ cells of the body can only be a small fraction of the vital reserve. We are now talking of the expenditure needed for the day. The previous day's energy was received that morning and by the time night set in, the person, though living in every sense of the term, felt too tired to carry on the activities of the body and the mind. Only the most essential functions continue inside, while the person sleeps. After that night's sleep and the next morning the organs are back with their quota of energy to conduct the next day's activity. This drama continues throughout life indicating that the life power is distributed from the vital reserve maintained for conducting the day's activity from morning till sleep. The energy that is given for the day's activity could be termed vitality or *jeevan shakti*.

The illusion

The proper supply of nutrients absorbed through the digested portion of food creates an illusion that the body has become energetic as mistakenly assumed that the food has 'imparted' energy to the body.

A tired organ is stimulated to activity through mild irritation occasioned by some so-called stimulant or tonic and this apparent increase in energy again creates an illusion that the body can be energised from outside.

A weak or overworked bowel, unable to discharge its functions, is irritated by a purgative or laxative when that bowel is compelled to throw out the irritant laxative along with faecal matter. This way, yet another illusion pervades to the effect that the bowel has been activated.

An emetic is given to a person and his stomach through irritation occasioned by that emetic, is forced to vomit out its contents; yet another illusion. The kidneys in a particular case, being very weak, are unable to effectively discharge their function, so a diuretic is administered. The diuretic occasions irritation in the kidney and the person urinates. It is believed by the concerned person that the drug has activated his kidneys; this is yet another illusion.

The world is full of such illusions. Action should be a normal physiological action not occasioned through irritation by any kind of external substance. Every forced action is like inflicting violence on the constitution. Submission to a system of medication is akin to declaring a war on the human constitution.

The sooner the above truth is realised the better it would be for mankind. Let every action of every organ be a normal physiological action. Even where a person has become diseased due to his adoption of unhygienic habits of living, some physiological action will be there. Let every action be within the available physiological limit.

An immature person may consider a disease as having been thrust upon him by some inimical force. But if the law of cause and effect is taken into account, this perverted view of disease can no longer be sustained. No one in the world wants to be diseased; all human beings desire to remain healthy all through life but for this, one has to, logically, stick to the practice of healthy living. There is no way other than this to remain healthy. It is a pity of pities that this basic truth is not accepted as the correct approach to fulfillment of man's innate desire to be healthy throughout life.

Man is endowed with intellect to enable him to think clearly, analyse correctly and solve all problems that crop up in worldly life from time to time. Blind acceptance of an irrational theory is something which the intellect should never submit to.

There are good and evil forces acting on every human being; it is man's intellect which should clearly enable him to discern the truth fearlessly and reject what is untruth, what is unreal, what is opposed to Nature's laws. Whether man likes it or not, the evil forces will persist. But the sensible man should remain unaffected by them.

The evil forces referred to are nourished and sustained by vested interests in various fields. These vested interests take the help of scientific jargon and blare out their views forcefully throughout the world. Man is told that health is a highly technical subject, that disease is man's enemy planted in him by germs, viruses, microbes, and the like and that cure of the disease is also a technical art which an ordinary man cannot master.

As most men in the modern world are engaged in earning their livelihood and cannot afford to waste time on illness by resting at home, they meekly accept the 'findings' of vested interests and rush to the doctor to seek medical help.

Life and livelihood

Every man has to spend a major portion of his daily life in dealing with problems concerning his livelihood. But here one is tempted to ask: Of what avail is man's existence on this planet if he does not know how to live, what the problems of life are and how a deep probe into his health would help him lead a happy and holy life on this planet?

The advice of the Nature therapist to the troubled man of today is: *"So long as man does not care to devote even a little time every day to the most important question of health and healthy living, so long as he is all the time tense and worried about the problems of his livelihood (centred around acquiring more and more wealth) no help whatever can be rendered to him in keeping him disease-free. Hence, however baffling the problem of livelihood be, let man attend to the first and foremost duty of his, that is, to maintain at least normal physical and mental health and, if possible, make effort to improve his health level steadily, as the so-called 'successful life' without physical and mental health is totally meaningless. Let every man and every woman know what hygienic living is, how it is to be lived through the perverted times of the modern days and how each one can be free, totally free from chronic and destructive diseases."*

Worldwide efforts are being made by man to restore the ecological balance. Let man also attempt to keep his internal ecology balanced so that the life power can work towards health without let or hindrance. This is his first and foremost duty.

To be successful in this endeavour, every human being must totally understand the need for observing vital economy in daily life. It is the non-observance of this most important principle concerning human health that is responsible for the ever-increasing incidence of disease in the world.

Vital economy

Each human being, being a separate entity, must so channelise the expenditure of his vitality in daily life as not to waste that precious power on any non-essential, unwanted, unhygienic activity—physiological, physical, mental. This may appear to be difficult to adopt in daily life, but there is no alternative to it. It may appear to be difficult because what is advocated here is not quite in tune with the habits prevalent in the civilisation-oriented world of today.

As modern civilisation is 'guided' by vested interests, as each vested interest works against every other and as all vested interests advocate the leading of licentious life, the question of adopting vital economy appears far from possible.

Is not leading life in a diseased state with daily intake of drugs a very sad experience? And is it not time for man to boldly face the truth and solve the baffling health problems of today?

It is undoubtedly true that with the failure of the drug system in curing chronic and destructive diseases more and more people the world over are taking to Nature cure. But those who still persist with drug medication, should they not learn from the experience of those on whom the drug systems have already failed? Should they not turn to Nature cure before things worsen? To every one of them the author's appeal is: *"There is no alternative to Nature cure, that is, care of your body and care of your mind in the manner intended by Mother Nature, the giver, the maintainer of life and the real and only healer on earth."*

Every step/method that is in tune with the principle of 'vital economy' will qualify to be non-violent in the light of the detailed explanation given above. In other words, what is not vital economy will be in violation of the principle of non-violence.

Tips for promoting vital economy

- Learn to breathe better but within the limits of each one's bodily constitution. Let everyone do non-violent *pranayama*. Let him perfect to the extent possible the processes of breathing out, breathing in and external and internal retention of air. *Pranayama* should be done where there is no air pollution and preferably early in the morning, after clearing the bowels.

- Ensure external cleanliness by keeping the atmosphere around as clean as possible. But in maintaining such cleanliness one should strictly keep away from the use of all chemicals or patent products that may be there in many 'cleansing agents'.
- Maintain one's bodily posture by keeping the backbone in its proper position. Bending forward and continuing to do one's work for hours on end or resting on soft beds or using tight footwear or exerting undue pressure on the bones of the feet through use of high-heeled shoes, etc.
- A dress made of synthetic fibre would adversely upset the normal working of the skin. Wearing a tight dress over any part of the body would make it difficult for the skin to discharge its normal function of breathing. Clothing should be for comfort and according to the weather. Overdressing is as bad as, or worse than, overeating and should be curbed.

  In the modern society, employees working in different professions have to don 'uniforms' that are prescribed, however much they may be against the principles of healthy living. Let these people at least wear the natural dress when they are off duty. Let these people take air-bath and if possible, sunbath too, every day. Let them keep their skin clean, by not troubling it with ointments, chemicals, synthetic products and toilet soaps.
- To maintain the structural integrity of every organ and

keep every system functionally efficient, natural food is advisable. It should be taken as whole and fresh as possible and in moderate doses to the extent required.

Those who are ill must keep away from food to the extent advocated in this book, else health recovery would be practically impossible. The maxim that food is a tax on vitality, that food is not the source of energy must be clearly perceived by the health-seeker.

Whatever is consumed during the day as food should be fresh, should be whole and predominantly alkaline. Hence, when preparing the salad, or cooking different dishes, the wholeness of food, the freshness of food should be tampered only to the unavoidable minimum extent.

Frugality in eating is very important. Even when one is healthy, taking more than two meals a day amounts to violation of vital economy, as work and digestion do not go together and no one should work on a loaded stomach. Care should be taken to consume very light meals before or during work hours. The main meal of the day should be moderate, not heavy; it should contain plenty of raw vegetables and fruits and should be taken only after one's daily work is over. Moderation in eating is ensured by chewing each morsel of food as thoroughly as possible.

All unnatural foods like tinned, bottled, packed, preserved foods, etc. are best avoided as none of these is fresh and as they contain preservatives, synthetic colour and synthetic flavour added to them.

- Attitude towards one's daily work should be positive. Let not any person dislike or hate his work. Sincerity in doing one's daily work, devoting attention to every detail concerning it would help in toning up the nerves and glands in the body.

- Time for leisure and entertainment should be set aside after one's work routine to enable a person to relax physically and mentally. Let this time be spent in such hobbies or recreational activities as would not expose him to health hazards like radiation emanating from video games or television. If possible, such leisure time could best be utilised by engaging oneself in constructive activities concerning one's moral development.
- Stimulants, drugs, etc., however popular these may be in the society around, should be totally eliminated from one's daily programme of living and for conservation of vitality.
- Non-violence in the treatment programme for recovery/ improvement of health in patients should be carried out so as not to exert even the least violence on any organ of the body or mind.

  For instance, the water used in the enema should be the minimum, say 250 grams. Hot water should be avoided. Use of soap, glycerine, etc. in water is objectionable. The tube conveying water to the anus should not be more than 60 to 65 centimetres long. Similarly the water used in the spinal-bath, hip-bath, etc. should be as cool as bearable. Steam-bath must be avoided as application of steam over the skin involves violence. Violent massage also is not acceptable. *Pranayama* must be done non-violently. Air-baths should be taken in pleasantly cool air. Fasting should be done as per the needs of the patient and not violently. Measures like acupressure, acupuncture, magneto-therapy, etc. should not be resorted to as these provide only symptomatic relief violating the basic law of cause and effect.
- Total approach is advocated in the science of natural hygiene as it is health-oriented and good for adoption.

> But let no one take to only a single method and 'swear' by it, avoiding all others. What is needed is a total approach wherein all activities in a man's daily life allow the principle of 'vital economy' to run as the common thread through everyone of them. Let there be no negative attitude of mind. Let the treatment be done very carefully and understandingly.

At present those who adopt natural hygiene are few in number and in mathematical terms these form a small minority. Hence, the habits advocated in natural hygiene may even be misrepresented as unfashionable. However, as life is meant to be lived with the sole object of promoting physical and mental health and as any 'other' plan cannot achieve the sole object of life on earth, the philosophy of natural hygiene has to be imbibed by everyone.

what is *prana*?

The human body is so unique that the innate intelligence in each cell, each tissue, each organ and each system is so tuned as to achieve a noble purpose. The organs within the body of the human being are ever at work, each discharging its Nature-ordained function(s), each working for the welfare of the whole. The nervous system conveys energy to each and every part of the body enabling it to work effectively.

The well-knit organisation that the human body possesses, the symbiotic relationship among the different organs in the body, the somatic awareness that each living cell in the body possesses and the manner in which all the functions of the body are carried on in a well-regulated fashion — all these make a man sit up and wonder at the secret behind this engineering marvel! How many amongst us care to understand the secrets behind such a complex organisation?

Even in this scientific era, people do not care to devote even a little attention to understand the power behind life. Practically all essential activities in the human body are carried on involuntarily and that is why most people do not care to devote the needed attention. The tendency that as the energy that serves to keep all functions going in a clock-like manner is available 'free', everyone seems to take the matter lightly. No thought whatever is devoted to the continued proper maintenance and upkeep of the body that has been endowed by Nature on the human being.

Mistake not the body for a 'machine'. Available physiological facts may seem to indicate that almost every organ is working mechanically and that by some manipulation (either physical or chemical) here or there it may even be possible to regulate the working of the concerned organs to create a semblance of 'normal working'. Whereas every machine in the world requires some power (like electricity) from outside to work, the human body has its own power inside the body.

Serious thought has to be devoted by every health-seeker on the points mentioned below. It is *prana* and *prana* alone that can help in normalising the condition of the body even where it has become abnormal.

When in quite some cases there is an apparent breakdown inside this organisation, the 'problem' is sought to be tackled quite mechanically, as in the instances cited below:

- *Problem*: Is any 'acidity' felt in the stomach due to more secretion of hydrochloric acid?

  Solution: Neutralise it with alkaline mixtures.

- *Problem*: Is the appendix inflamed and the concerned person is 'troubled' by this development?

  Solution: Surgically remove the appendix.

- *Problem*: Is the blood pressure much more than normal?

  Solution: Reduce the blood pressure by the use of hypotensives.

- *Problem*: Is anyone having constipation?

  Solution: Use purgatives or laxatives or resort to colonic irrigation.

- *Problem*: Is there stone in the kidney or the gall bladder?

  Solution: Remove the stone surgically.
- *Problem*: Is tension being experienced by a person?

  Solution: Use tranquillisers.
- *Problem*: Is any pain being experienced in any part of the body?

  Solution: Use pain-killers.

The above methods are advocated under what is called the scientific approach in health care or medi-care. Very few go deep into the problem they face to find out the real cause of the particular disease condition they are experiencing.

Maintenance of body in the near ideal state presupposes the availability of the requisite energy needed for the purpose.

To enable a patient to cure himself radically and to re-establish normalcy inside his body also presupposes the availability of the requisite energy inside the body. The one question that is to be probed into is: 'Where lies this energy inside? Can this energy be transmitted into the body from somewhere outside in any manner?' The approach adopted by natural hygiene enables man to undertake this probe.

Mistaking the body as a machine

Let us before explaining the stand of natural hygiene on the above vital issue, first clarify that the human body may look like a perfect machine and the organs therein may work like a machine. But it will be totally wrong and opposed to Nature's laws to look upon it mechanically.

Possibly most people do not recognise that the incidence of what is known as iatrogenic disease is due to the drugs employed earlier. In other words, these are the after-effects and side-effects of the drugs consumed earlier.

The very science which advocates the use of such remedies also lists the after-effects and side-effects in extenso. Can this 'mode' of treatment be deemed to be a rational one? Let everybody seriously ponder over this question. Does not the use of different drugs result in sapping the vitality of the person as time goes by? No one seems to worry about this question.

Let us for a moment put away the problem of the diseased person and look at a fairly healthy person. Is he taking steps to rationally understand what is maintaining his health and how he can progressively improve his health level in times to come? Here again the answer is in the negative, for science is in fact unaware of the only energy that is behind the working of the human system.

On the other hand, food is said to be the source of energy. Even people consuming foods in accordance with calorie tables are falling ill or steadily becoming weaker and all attempts to 'energise' man through the intake of food end in utter failure. Where energy fails, stimulants or so-called tonics of one kind or the other are taken in by the modern man. Different stimulants seem to achieve immediate results. But their continued use results in steady vital depletion.

Let no one mistake the above statement as coming from a person who condemns science. Science as such cannot be condemned. The adoption of scientific temper of mind is very much needed. But to adopt the scientific temper to understand issues fundamentally, to solve problems rationally, one must have all the needed background data.

Every human being has life power or *prana shakti* that is behind the working of each living cell in the body. The oxidation of food occurring in the digestive system may 'resemble' energy, but to mistake this as the energy that is behind the bodily working tantamounts to the negation of the existence of life power inside man.

Whatever the 'claims' of the modern science, the human body cannot be energised by any mechanical means either from within the body or by any other means from outside. If only such a measure could be practically put into operation, it should be possible to avert even death; it should be possible to energise a vitally depleted person. Science can never succeed in such attempts for life power inside man is super physical, super chemical in nature and nothing like it can be manufactured or produced by man anywhere in the world.

The adoption of the scientific temper of mind can reveal the truth behind the statement contained in the preceding paragraph.

What is *prana*?

The vital energy or *prana shakti* can be a mystery far beyond the understanding of modern man. Ancient sages were able to understand the mystery through contemplation in their inner laboratories after cleansing their minds and hearts of the weaknesses, which the ordinary man was exposed to even in the good old days.

The various physiological functions all the time going on in a living organism are due to the presence of *prana shakti* in every cell/tissue/organ. This *prana shakti* cannot be X-rayed or taken out of the body and analysed or subjected to any so-called scientific scrutiny. Whenever forces like electricity, magnetism, etc., act, though understood to some extent by modern science and put to practical use through scientific instruments, what their real shape is and how these are made available to man by Nature continues to be a mystery. When even these are a mystery, how much more mysterious should be the power *prana* operating through living organism? Any attempt to define any of the functions of *prana* would tend to be incorrect in some way or the other, for, it is beyond our understanding.

Yet for the limited purpose of having some basic knowledge of how to keep oneself healthy through sensible self-control over all the organs that constitute the human body as also over the mind and the real *indriyas* operating from the inner body or *antahkaran* (the sense organs in the gross body visible to the human being are just receptacles and nothing more), an attempt is being made here to express what is really inexpressible in words.

To communicate the different physical functions of *prana* inside the living body through the five subdivisions of *prana* (into *prana, apana, vyana, udana* and *samana*) are indicated below. In reality *prana* is one but when carrying out the different functions it assumes other names. When carrying out one group of functions, its name continues to be *prana.*

There are references at various places in the *Vedic* lore on what *prana* is and how it functions through the living body. Given below is a brief description of how different functions in the human body are directed, controlled and regulated by *prana* (in its various facets). What are known as *apana, vyana, udana,* and *samana* are also facets of *prana shakti* and these names are given to *prana* when the functions vary according to needs.

- ***Prana*** is that facet of life power which ensures the much needed heat (known as the normal bodily temperature) is evenly distributed all through the body, ensuring the proper functioning of the heart all through life and enabling man to see through his eyes, to hear through his ears and to breathe and smell through his nose.
- ***Apana*** is that facet of life power which ensures the proper

functioning of the different eliminatory organs as also the power that is behind the functioning of the generative organs. In other words, *apana* is the power that controls elimination of waste matter from the body and ensures that where need be, waste is eliminated through channels other than eliminatory organs to ensure internal sanitation. This is what is meant by elimination of matter through acute disease or through healing crisis.

Apana is also that facet of life power which is behind the virility of the reproductive organ. By sensible control over the functioning of the reproductive organ through the practice of *brahmacharya* (self-control through all the five organs, i.e. *jnanendriyas* of perception), a lot of vital power is saved, ensuring conservation of vitality inside the body through one's lifetime and see to it that the progeny is bestowed with good physical and mental health.

- ***Vyana*** is that facet of the life power, which, through the heart pervades the whole body, seeing to it that the nerve energy needed for performing various activities through various organs in the body is made available at the appropriate time to the concerned organs. *Vyana* is again that facet of life power that regulates proper circulation of blood through the veins and arteries throughout the whole body. It is said that *vyana* controls the subtle body, which means that *vyana* ensures the proper functioning of intellect or *buddhi*, the power of discrimination or *viveka*, etc.

- ***Udana*** is that facet of life power which is located at that vital point in the gullet where the respiratory tract and the digestive tract part from each other, ensuring that no food or drink enters the respiratory tract, adversely affecting man's ability to breathe in and breathe out.

- ***Samana*** is that facet of life power, which ensures that the nutrients derived from the digested food are distributed to the different systems and different organs in the body according to their needs. In other words, this is that facet of life power that is behind the law of vital distribution, day after day on a daily basis. This is what is also known as *jeevan shakti*.

Prana, which cannot be produced inside the body by any action of man or taken in by him from any external source by his will, is understood as the life power inherent in him since birth. However, as no action can be executed without a corresponding expenditure of power in every action of man — physical or mental, internal or external — vital energy is spent in the day from that made available to man through his *jeevan shakti* . If a person violates the laws of health and takes to unhygienic living habits compelling the *jeevan shakti* to overdraw from the vital reserve (such overdrawal is permitted by life to avert the catastrophe that might occur otherwise), the person concerned is well on the road towards vital depletion in the not so far future.

As conservation of *prana* is the only manner through which a person could live long and healthy without any disease, common sense decrees that the principle of vital economy should be followed in daily life as scrupulously as possible. There were and there are instances where persons leading a licentious life and adopting unhygienic habits were afflicted by chronic or destructive disease. These instances are but warnings to mankind to lead a well-regulated life to the extent practicable.

Objective before the health-seeker

Wisdom decrees that man should, therefore, avoid falling victim to chronic and destructive diseases that invite premature death. He should regulate his daily activities in such a manner that entails the least possible expenditure of his vitality in every action of his.

The enlightened sages of yore helped mankind with knowledge relating to the working of the *prana shakti* in his body. And the modern sage, Acharya Lakshmana Sarma has worked out all the details as to how the health-seeker can economise on the expenditure of his vitality while discharging his duties during the course of his worldly life.

Death is inevitable for everyone that is born. Let that point of death come not through disease and suffering at a premature age. Let it come at a ripe old age (without any disease) as a result of the slow and steady depreciation that inevitably occurs in the human body. Observance of the principle of vital economy will ensure longevity and health upto a ripe old age.

We have so far learnt that vitality available day after day for enabling man to function effectively within as also efficiently in the world outside is drawn from the vital reserve of *prana shakti* within and having recognised that health (a positive state of well-being of the body and the mind, wherein the occurrence of any chronic or destructive disease is totally impracticable) and longevity fully depend upon the frugal expenditure of the *jeevan shakti* in one's daily life. Every sane man/woman should follow the principle of vital economy in one's daily life.

The source of *prana*

The question that may arise is—wherefrom has this power been made available to all persons? The obvious answer is—from the Creator who has created, is creating and will be creating in human beings.

Let us look beyond *prana shakti* to find out what lies there.

The power that is known as *prana shakti* (with its variant *jeevan shakti*) is just like the power available in a house inside a building. Such power is made available to all the buildings from a central powerhouse, which is the Supreme Being or *paratattva,* who keeps the world show going on. So the modern man must realise that he owes the power within him to that power beyond.

As the human being is a triple unit of body, mind and spirit and as the functions of the body and the mind are vitalised by the soul or *jeevatma* through the medium of *prana shakti,* the health-seeker must realise and after so realising transform his way of life as not to waste his vital power through any physical or mental activities of dubious nature as far as possible. Not only is the personality concerned enriched, he can enrich so many people around him. Such is the power derived by practical observance of this principle of vital economy. The *Kathopanishad* clearly states: *"Not by* prana, *not by* apana *does any mortal live, but it is by some other on which these two depend that the mortals live."*

Prana is one of the names of God as given in the *Vishnu sahasranama,* the thousand names of Lord Vishnu in the *Mahabharata.* Still another name of Lord is given therein is *Pranadah,* the giver of *prana* to every being. Sri Shankarabhagawatpada, who is venerated as the incarnation or *avatar* of Lord Siva, refers to the Lord as the *prana* of *pranas.*

The author quotes this here just to impress on the reader that a rigorous observance of the principle of vital economy is tantamount to the worship of the Supreme Being. When along with the observance of this principle in the daily life, one also recognises the spiritual meaning of it in depth, the very personality of the human being as it were, gets electrified.

That this vital power so essential for the health and well-being of man can be conserved and by so conserving it to the extent possible, man can have health and longevity while alive is stressed in all scriptures the world over. Almost every scripture declares that the happiness and prosperity of man depends on the practice of virtues like serenity, sincerity, simplicity, veracity, magnanimity, charity, generosity, purity, etc. in his daily life. These virtues could rightly be termed as super nutrients, far more needed for the health and well-being of man than the nutrients given through food to the body.

In other words, unless and until man is wise enough to recognise his spiritual needs and sincere enough to supply these needs in a determined manner, ideal health or near ideal health cannot be achieved. It may be argued by some that in this scientific era of ours this suggestion of mine is tantamount to taking mankind back to the first century B.C. This 'charge' is due to ignorance in realising that the laws governing human health were, are and will remain the same all through time. These are eternal, immutable and inviolable.

Let us maintain all that is good in this scientific era (with its inventions and technologies) with the spirit of good life that forms the essence of natural hygiene. This could bring in a utopia, a heaven on earth. Let there be a civilisation without suffering, at the mental and physical levels.

Let every act of man in his day be done in the right spirit, in the right form and at the right place. Let every act be deemed as worship of God. The author has no doubt whatsoever that even in the modern world abounding in rationalists and atheists, it is quite possible for man to live in the manner indicated. Let our lives enlighten the sceptic that it is the *prana shakti* in him that makes him live in the world.

successfully piloting of one's life

The term 'successful living' is normally used to indicate the attainment of a good standard of education (technical or non-technical); engaging oneself in some money-earning activity; getting a life partner and running after sensual pleasures; increase in one's desires for luxuries to a limitless extent; hopping from one end of the globe to the other; travelling on high speed jets and keeping oneself so 'busy' as to find no time even for eating or rest.

Everyone wants to be 'successful' in life and each one is frantic in this mad race. That mad race for political power and for establishment of 'business empires' is also for the obvious purpose of achieving what has been outlined in the preceding paragraph.

The moot question is: Are these 'successful' people physically and mentally healthy? Are they free from tension any time? Are they able to sleep well and get up afresh the next morning? Are they really happy? Do they not have to indulge in rivalry, competition, double-dealing, etc. in relation to others around them? Are they not lacking satisfaction in life? Are they really happy with their lot?

A probe into these questions will reveal that most people are suffering from chronic diseases, carrying some pills, potions and powders in their pockets all the time; they are ever tense; they are mentally dissatisfied with their lot; they do not know how to 'escape' from the quagmire they are in; they get along in their lives with the help of stimulants, sedatives and the like; and even their family life leaves them dissatisfied.

The *maya* (the power of illusion) that is enveloping every immature man, makes most other men and women, who are not successful enough to make as much money in life, jealous of the so-called successful people and this jealousy makes their lives as miserable as that of the successful ones.

I want to assure the reader that I am not presenting a dismal picture of the prevailing situation. There is no harm in man aspiring to have plenty of money and property. There is no harm in aspiring for political power or in establishing powerful business houses. But everyone of these should be sought for a noble purpose. The motive must be good, unmixed with evil or selfishness. In my view, the person who does not even care to know the secret behind the maintenance of physical and mental health, the secret of leading a tension-free life, cannot be said to be living successfully, whatever his so-called 'achievement' in the world may be.

- He is a successful man who feels a sense of satisfaction all the time and who leads his life guided by noble principles.
- He is a successful man who carries out all his activities calmly, composedly, enjoying a stillness of mind (which he owes to his philosophical outlook on life).
- He is a successful man who helps his fellow-beings and does not exploit them.
- He is a successful man who, whatever his economic status in life, stands head and shoulders above everyone around.
- He is a successful man who cares for the welfare of the

members of his family, cares for them in the correct sense of the term and bestows enough attention on the development of character in his children.

- He is a successful man whose guidance is sought by people not well placed in life materially.

How many from among the modern people satisfy the criteria set above? No joy whatever can be derived by engaging in some routine work in some corner of the world just for the purpose of feeding oneself. One must have an ideal in life: A noble ideal to be achieved through pursuit of a disciplined way of life. Each one of us can go on expanding and expanding limitlessly one's ability to be of service to mankind. Each one of us is capable of expanding worthwhile knowledge and employing it for benefiting the society. Each is capable of developing good virtues in one's daily life, the possession of which could make him the richest man in the world. Let money be earned but not at the cost of honesty, not at the cost of virtuous living.

What goodwill is to business, good manners are to every man. Even as business cannot thrive without goodwill, man cannot successfully pilot through life without good manners.

To be able to successfully pilot through life one should, besides having good education, financial standing, a social status and the like, also have

- good health all through life;
- a sense of humility in the personality;
- receptivity to the teachings of elders in the society;
- ability to withstand the terrific shock given often by people in modern society;
- capacity to stand aloof from the rest when it comes to

question of sticking to one's principles, which he holds dear to his life.

Natural hygiene can help man

Having outlined the criteria that ought to guide man to live purposefully in the somewhat troubled modern world, let me clarify that all this could be achieved by following natural hygiene, based upon the eternal, immutable and inviolable laws that govern the physical and mental health of man.

Natural hygiene represents a way of life with a sensible philosophy underlying it. If principles of natural hygiene are adopted by a healthy individual, his health level would progressively go up. If these principles are adopted by unhealthy persons, even their health level would go up and with improved health level, they would be radically cured. As most people in modern days take to natural hygiene only for curing their diseases, this system is popularly called Nature cure, a name which we accept rather reluctantly.

Natural hygiene has no place for the use of remedies whatsoever. To advocate the use of a remedy for a particular disease is tantamount to a fragmentary approach in dealing with the problem of disease. Every habit in life has to be transmuted into a hygienic habit. The very discipline involved in switching to this life could make man happy, healthy and holy.

The objective

Are you a health seeker? Do you want to radically cure your disease? Do not adopt a fragmentary approach—the approach advocated in different systems of medication. Each of these systems prescribes only remedies for getting symptomatic relief. These remedies cannot improve one's level of health. To advocate the use of any remedy, to employ a remedy to get over the problem temporarily is in a sense an act of escapism.

Rightly the science of natural hygiene is totally against every type of medication for sound and firm reasons. To enable one to gain fully through natural hygiene, one must have a thorough knowledge of the fundamentals of this science of health. The health-seeker should first and foremost understand these fundamentals in depth, be convinced of the soundness of approach advocated therein and then he can achieve his goal of a near ideal state of health. It may however by noted that attainment of an ideal state is somewhat impracticable with so much of air pollution, water pollution, soil pollution, noise pollution, etc. around us. Even with these very disturbing circumstances, one can enjoy a near ideal state of health through natural hygiene, by the readiness on the part of the health-seeker to submit himself to the dictates of Mother Nature.

Having stressed the need for a clear knowledge of fundamentals let me stress upon one more vital point: Let not the health-seeker just take one or two suggestions made in natural hygiene and practise these while neglecting the rest. What is needed is a total approach. A mere morning walk cannot make one healthy; merely doing *asanas* and *pranayama* cannot make one healthy; taking raw salad in the day and at night cannot make one healthy. I would like to stress upon all health-seekers that adoption of a total approach is what is required for achievement of the objective.

We have already taken birth in this world with so many disadvantages around. Maybe what is termed as civilisation is openly advocating some of the disabling agents and methods, but as we may not have the ability to rectify the situation satisfactorily, we have to chart out a path for ourselves wherein, while living in civilised society, we remain unaffected by it. But let us take the noble resolve of living in this world of civilisation without any suffering whatever. Let the slogan be: 'Be civilised without suffering'!

prarabdha sans suffering

It is an undeniable fact that every person must go through the consequences of all his actions—good or bad, now (i.e. within a reasonable time) or later. In fact, it is this that has led to the formulation of many of the principles of ethics and morality current in society. The division of one's actions either belongs to virtue or to sin and the exhortations of wise men are that one should follow *dharma* or righteousness in all his actions— physical, mental, verbal—and resist from committing acts of sin.

All this pattern of thought current the world over from time immemorial is logical and anyone who thinks that he can with impunity commit vicious acts and can escape punishment is perhaps living in his own mental paradise.

What is popularly deemed as fear of God is only fear of consequences. God is not an unkind power imposing punishment on some people. What is expressed by the phrase 'fear of God' is perhaps none other than what is clearly specified in *Manu Smriti's* dictum:

"Dharma *punishes the person that violates the order and* dharma *protects the individual who goes in accordance with the established order."*

All that is stated above is quite in tune with that eternal law—the law of cause and effect. But what puzzles man is: Why is it that people who are leading a principled life by sticking to the performance of virtue are suffering from penury in their lives? Why is it that even some of their basic needs are not getting satisfied, and conversely, how is it that many people leading an unprincipled life are literally rolling in money and 'enjoying' plenty of physical comfort? These very questions seem to raise doubts on the applicability of the law of cause and effect.

There is what is known as the law of land prevalent in each country. Each of these laws has a penalty chapter, which would apply to those who violate the provisions of the concerned law. The law provides the extent to which penalty can be imposed upon the violator by those who are responsible for administering justice. Those that follow the principles of the law are 'protected' by the very law.

A person committs a heinous murder and absconds forever. The law is not able to punish him as he is untraceable. Has the law of cause and effect been set at naught in this case?

Another person commits an unsocial act of a very serious type, but the concerned man-made law with loopholes in it cannot punish him, for the loopholes in the law declare that he cannot be punished. Here again, has the law of cause and effect been annulled? It can never be.

Indian philosophy tells man that his present birth is but a link in the long chain of births that he had had earlier. But here again many modern people do not seem to understand this and seem to question its veracity.

Here are some problems/issues to be rolled over in one's mind:

- Why is it that two brothers and one sister born to the same parents have their different peculiar attitudes and have quite different experiences in their personal lives?
- How is it that a great genius is born to parents with very little education and very few material achievements? Why

is it that such persons of exceptional talents not equally recognised in the world at large?

Such questions can be raised *ad infinitum*. But there is in every language in the world, a word meaning 'destiny', which provides the answer to this issue. Each language has words of wisdom in it. Destiny is one such word. And, understanding what this means will unveil the puzzles that baffle modern mankind who do not have any faith in the theory of rebirth.

Does life end at death?

The laws codified in so many countries in the world may hold that as a person is dead, the cases against him pending in the courts have to be closed. But in the court of Mother Nature with Nature, as Chief Justice, presiding over the court (along with Justice Rightness, Justice Goodness, Justice Virtue and Justice Fairness as the other members of the judiciary) and functioning all the time unerringly, the cases pending against a person at death are never closed. Nature holds sway over man even beyond death.

The world over children are born every second. All may have the physical human frame but are their minds not different? Is it not seen that in spite of the same type of education, children in later lives flower as youth, each having a different personality? A few of them are 'gifted'. A few develop into poets and poetesses. A few choose to get into drinking and dancing. A few take to stealing, double dealing, and such other methods. Such unexplainable changes in persons are seen even among brothers/sisters/cousins belonging to the same family. Such questions raise more mysteries.

The fact is that each child born in this world has a vast background unknown to it and unknown to others in the world. And as this background varies from one child to the other, the children grow into different personalities.

The past

This past is the load of *karma* (what each language in the world chooses to call as 'destiny') on the back of each child that is born. This is known as the *prarabdha karma,* the word *prarabdha* meaning that part of *karma,* which has started 'taking effect'. This term indicates that there is a part of the load of *karma,* which has not started taking effect, which is kept in the account of the concerned individual. But this load of *karma* too has to be cleared some time later in future births. This is termed as *sanchita karma,* the word *sanchita* meaning that the load is being kept in reserve; it is not operative during the present birth.

As the child takes birth and grows to pass through childhood, adolescence, youth and old age, he has necessarily to indulge in actions, good and bad. Nature has designed that no one can be free from action. These good and bad actions done by a person go on accumulating, not yielding results even immediately in this birth. But as no action done at a time can be kept away without the person experiencing the fruit thereof, this new burden of *karma* goes on accumulating. This is known as *agami karma* in Indian philosophy.

It is the *prarabadha karma* that has led to the present birth. *Prarabdha karma* is *karma* which has started taking its effect and no one, not even a person who has discovered the ultimate secret and gone up high in the spiritual ladder, can get away from the *prarabdha karma* allotted to him at the time of his birth.

Let us now see whether there are permitted and sensible ways to clear off the *sanchita karma,* the load of which is far heavier than that of *prarabdha*. Let us also simultaneously find out if it is practicable to ensure that the *agami karma* of man in his present birth is rendered fruitless, not capable of being added to the burden of *karma*. If these two loads can be cleared as per the guidance given to man by sages, what is left out is the *prarabdha karma*. And even here, with the proper application of one's power of discrimination and through the development of virtuous qualities, this could be passed through with practically no suffering in this world.

What has been stated in the preceding paragraph is not, as many in the modern world may seem to suppose, for a selected few—the blessed ones; it is for all. Wisdom decrees that the eternal truths at the back of the theory of *karma* have to be understood by every person—each person who takes birth in the world must be enriched by the understanding of these 'eternal truths' and on getting the requisite enlightenment, start acting on the right lines. My plea to everyone would be: "Do not dismiss this with contempt."

Life is not a bed of roses in every case. This everyone knows. To many people it happens to be misery unlimited, with problems staring at them all the time. When this is the actual case, would it not be worthwhile to know how one can ensure that this birth of ours could be the last birth—there being no further rebirth?

However much and however easily the rich heritage (the common property of all) is divulged to the people living in the modern times, there appear to be two serious blinding factors that blind the vision of the modern man to truth. One such blinding factor is what is known as 'science'. When man is possessed by this blinding factor, his intellect tells him: 'All this is unscientific.' Let them ponder—Can science find out the answers to all the puzzles? There are a million and odd puzzles which due to lack of space do not find place in this chapter. Let those overpowered by the world of science ponder over these questions seriously, deeply, with all possible inner contemplation. Where physics melts into the thin air of metaphysics, is there not something beyond it? Can physics reveal it? How is it that parallel lines, which should not at all touch each other, meet at infinity?

The other one that blinds many is 'materialism'. Many in the modern world are blinded by the belief that what matters in life is monetary affluence. Here are some questions which require to be seriously pondered and reflected upon: Granted that monetary affluence favours particular persons, does even one of them have a sense of satisfaction in life, good sleep and good digestion? Are such persons mentally calm, composed, looking at their different problems sensibly and critically? Are they free from tension all the time? Do they have even an inkling of what is beyond life?

The author is sure that those blinded by science and materialism to the total exclusion of the eternal truths enshrined in the cultural background would turn dumbfounded when they reach this dead end. Perhaps this is a stage where even a U-turn would be impossible.

Let 'science' be there, let 'materialism' be there; but let it be realised that these are not the be all and end all.

Clearing the *agami karma* load

That each one born in this world has to go through different experiences, some sweet, some sour and some even bitter during his/her life, is known to all. Even brothers, sisters, cousins brought up in the same environment and under somewhat similar circumstances in their early lives have varied experiences, each different from every other. The mental make-up of each person varies, sometimes even one is antagonistic to another. What is the basic factor shaping the experience of each one in this world?

However much one may put in serious efforts to make his/her future happy and prosperous, destiny has its own way of making the person submit to it willingly or unwillingly.

The whole question bristling with problems all around has been analysed and thrashed out by the wise men of ancient India. Their probe has brought up the theory of *karma* as the basic cause for the different experiences of different persons in their lives. Here, in brief is a summary, the sum and substances of their findings in this regard.

The actions, which each *jeeva* (living being) in this world engages itself upon, naturally produce reactions/effects, which later turn into fresh actions producing further reactions/effects. This unending cycle goes on. Life on earth being limited to a few years (may be fifty, sixty or seventy) or in some cases even far less, it is practically not possible to clear off all the *karma*. Hence, the load of *karma* uncleared goes on accumulating in each *jeeva's* account. But as all has to be cleared totally, each *jeeva* has to be reborn taking some 'body' or the other.

When the *jeeva* is reborn, Nature assigns to it its portion taken from the accumulated load of *karma* and assigns that small portion of *karma* to be cleared in that life. This is what is termed as *prarabdha karma,* that is, *karma* which has started taking effect during the course of that life.

Whatever is left in the accumulated load of *karma* (to be cleared off in the numerous rebirths, which each *jeeva* is to take in future) is termed as *sanchita karma.* This load of *karma* is not operative during the present life but is kept in account.

During the course of the present life, each *jeeva* is all the time engaged in some action or the other, each of which produces its own reaction/effect. This series of *karma* being done in the present birth is known as *agami karma.*

Of the three, *prarabdha* has started taking effect. No one on earth can annul or put it off. *Sanchita* is inoperative during the present birth. But one has to take future births, which cannot be avoided. As for *agami karma,* there is a way, so the wise men of yore say to see to it that these are not added to the load of *sanchita karma* so that the *agami karma* can be rendered 'ineffective'. By taking this wise step the person would not be adding to his misery further. What is the method suggested? Behind every action done by a person there ought to be a motive. Though the action done by different persons may be the same, the motive of each person doing it may differ from one another. Motives depend on the peculiar attitude each one has towards life and its problems. Normally each person doing an action is doing it in order to derive some benefit from such action. The idea of agency (what is termed as *kartrtva bhava* in Indian philosophy) is prominent in each of man's actions. Simultaneously with it there is a 'desire' in the mind of each person to enjoy the fruits of his actions, and this is termed as *bhoktrtva bhava* in the Indian philosophy. So long as the idea of agency and the desire to enjoy the fruits of action 'possess' man's mind, that long he is bound by every action of his. Unendingly the load of *sanchita karma* will be added on.

Our ancient seers say: "*Whether you like it or not, you have to be doing some action or the other all the time in your life.*" Do the action, but will it not be wise on your part to see that these actions do not bind you in future? Please realise that it is possible to do an action without the *kartrtva bhava.* Can't you realise that you are being 'impelled' by your *prarabdha karma* to do an action? Why not consider yourself as an instrument of destiny? Why do you have the idea of agency in you?

Similarly, each one of your actions is again impelled by your *prarabdha,* without any desire to enjoy the fruits thereof.

Do your *karma* but renounce the fruits of all such actions. This renunciation of the desire to enjoy the fruits of your action is a form of the science of yoga known as *karma yoga.* You do not stand to lose anything in this life by adopting this spirit of renunciation. It is not as if you would not get anything out of actions. But whatever comes out of it as its effect is (taken sportingly) will not affect you emotionally in any manner.

The adoption of the above attitude towards every action impelled by your *prarabdha* will so change your inner personality that you will literally be like the water on the lotus leaf. Your *karma* would not have the least effect on your inner personality and you will not have any desire whatsoever for enjoying the result from any action. If you adopt this attitude, *agami karma* would not accumulate. Thus you have ensured that there is no further addition to the *sanchita karma* kept in your account at the time of your birth.

Sanchita karmas **too get fried**

If any person has adopted the attitude described above, Nature with all her grace cancels all *sanchita karma* in the person's account just as fried seed cannot sprout again. All the *sanchita karma* get fried.

Agami karmas are made fruitless, the *sanchita karmas* have got fried and the concerned person has practically no burden of *karma* on him. Only the *prarabdha,* which has somehow to be cleared, is there on him. Even towards these *karma* his attitude is sportive. He goes through the experiences literally unaffected by them. He does his worldly work; he mixes with people of different temperaments. All this can affect him neither this way nor that way. Having reached this stage the person concerned keeps his mind calm, unruffled. Though the *prarabdha karma* might impose some suffering on him, he does not get mentally upset himself. He undergoes the experience as happily as a *satyagrahi* cheerfully accepts the term of imprisonment imposed on him.

Having explained in brief how one should pilot his *prarabdha* plane through the summit of wisdom, I have to tell patients at present suffering from chronic and destructive disease and who are taking to science of natural hygiene for recovering health, "Please do not commit the mistake of engaging yourself in unhygienic actions and put the blame on your so-called *prarabdha*. Live hygienically. Adopt sane and safe ways of recovering your health. Do self-surrender (*aatma samarpana*) to Mother Nature. Let not the minor sufferings imposed on you by your prarabdha unnerve you. Take it as a *satyagrahi* should take his travails sportingly. Suffering of any type gone through cheerfully purifies the personality, ennobles the personality. Do not, like many others around you, go on blaming your *prarabdha* if anything untoward happens. Pray to God that you should have the courage to develop the spirit of renunciation of the fruits of actions, which is extolled by Lord Sri Krishna as the yoga of *karma phala tyaga* to uplift man. It is also possible for ordinary persons to do all this."

Having stressed on the need for a clear knowledge of fundamentals, the author stresses upon one more vital point: *"Let not the health-seeker just take one or two of the suggestions made in natural hygiene and practise these alone, neglecting the rest. What is most needed is a total approach pasted over one's hat that a mere morning walk cannot make one healthy.* Merely doing asanas *and* pranayama *cannot ensure good health; merely taking raw salad in the day and at night cannot make one healthy."* The author would like to stress upon all health-seekers that adoption of the total approach is what is required for achievement of the objective.

total approach

Everyone in the world wants to enjoy ideal health but the fact remains that health appears to 'elude' most people. Why? The answer that follows to this question will reveal the truth in all its splendour.

In the days of yore man had no problems whatsoever. He had everything in the most natural form and by and large, his instincts guided him to eat only when he was hungry, to rest when he was tired, to keep away from strain and stress (which used to be rarely there) and to lead his life in an atmosphere where man-made complications and problems did not entail stress on his life. The situation today happens to be unfortunately at the other extreme. Man's natural instincts appear to have become perverted. Air is polluted and water too. The tension which is a by-product of man's eagerness to take to high pressure living in tune with the urge of modern civilisation, the almost total absence of need on man's part to have any worthwhile physical activity—these are only some, not all, of puzzles and riddles created by man around him in the modern world. No wonder that diseases are rampant almost everywhere.

Here too, instead of tackling the real cause of the disease, man goes on indulging in symptomatic treatment and 'corrective' surgery. Such is the dismal picture of man's health in modern days.

Quite a few persons thought of escaping from the web of

life and taking to natural hygiene. Though they found some relief through the adoption of the new approach of natural hygiene, they could not 'fully' benefit. Where lay the snag?

For centuries mankind had got addicted to the view that the medicine man (who had mastered the art) was very necessary for curing a patient. Most people happen to run after a 'medicine man', as they do not consider natural hygiene an alternative system of medicine on par with other systems of medication. In other words, they do not recognise the truth fully and fall into the clutches of some other system they see before them.

The remedy mindedness–a curse

So long as man equates the apparent effect of a remedy with a radical cure of the original disease (whatever the nomenclature of disease be), there is no hope for mankind. The fact that many people are taking to natural hygiene in modern days and even deriving some benefit out of it does not gladden the mind of the writer for practically everyone of these happens to be remedy minded.

Psychologically speaking, the one who seeks remedies for his problems is an escapist inasmuch as he is unwilling to face his problem, to study his problem in depth and find the solution therefor by himself. And a person who is possessed by this 'demon' of escapism does never recognise the truth that his problem can be solved.

Not an alternative system of medicine

The ancient *Ayurveda* which was in its prime purity in ancient days in India has lost its lustre and become a glass piece (apparently shining) now.

Back in those earliest days when the population in the world was very sparse, man lived in isolated hamlets, huts and houses. Each one had to look after the satisfaction of all his needs, as there was no organised profession in the society then. And under such circumstances each person was caring for his own health. The science of *Ayurveda* in its prime purity was present and each person was his own doctor. The health problems were practically few.

What was the original *Ayurveda* that existed in those days? We may get an idea of it from the most ancient work, *Ayurveda Sutram* (in Sanskrit). This rare work has been published by the University of Mysore and even now those having knowledge of Sanskrit might peruse the work. It talks of natural hygiene, as we understand it today. As in course of time, the population grew and as man began to settle in small towns and villages, the need for creating occupational classification in society was felt. Various occupations (namely, masons, carpenters, potters, teachers, etc.) became established in the society. The persons in each of these professions served the others in exchange for the supply of their basic needs of living like foodgrains, clothes, etc. from others. This was a social development of a right type.

But a few people in society came up and said: "We shall be your doctors caring for your health and every one of you need not take the trouble of understanding *Ayurveda*." Society got divided into two groups: (1) the medicine men and (2) the others. In the initial stages no one fell ill and thus the medicine men had no work to do. Hence, they began to make science as complicated as possible and created an impression that everyone could not learn it. As time rolled by, more and more illnesses set in the society and the *Ayurveda* as is being practised today is what has come out of this untoward development in society, which started centuries ago.

Though lip service is being paid to words like 'hygiene' and 'health', mankind as a whole seems to be in the dark and even those with knowledge of the science of Nature cure happen to present it as an alternative system of medicine in a complicated manner. This is because many of them happen to be professionals in their line—prototypes of those earliest *Ayurvedic* doctors who did not want all the people to be healthy but wanted patients to serve their (doctor's) own ends.

What is popularly known as Nature cure is nothing more than what Acharya Lakshmana Sarma termed as 'life natural'—the adoption of that mode of life which has because designed by Mother Nature. Some followers in the West term this as natural hygiene or the science of health based on Nature's laws of health which are irrefutable. They could have called it simply 'hygiene' but to distinguish it from spurious hygiene, particularly today when poisons and medicaments are used, the Western followers termed it as natural hygiene.

Are you the health-seeker?

If the above question is posed before us, the reply will be in affirmative. Well, your health totally depends upon your having a clean bloodstream, proper blood circulation with structural integrity of every organ in near ideal state and proper functional efficiency of every system (like respiratory system, the digestive system, etc.) in good condition. Why not remind yourself of the truth that the conditions obtaining inside your body are entirely your own creation depending upon your habits of living? No one can make you ill if you are determined to be well and no one can give you health from outside if you are living wrongly. Why not remind yourself of these basic truths?

The above basic requirement of health can be had only if your body and mind are cared for as Nature intends you to care for them, for after all, the human body is designed by

Nature and Nature has complete suzerainty over all the functions and activities inside the organism. In other words, no mechanical manipulation from outside, no mechanical contrivances, etc. can help to 'normalise' the condition within.

Why not recognise this truth? Natural hygiene is a codification of the concerned natural laws of health. This is not an alternative system of medicine but a way of life to be followed by every sane individual in the world.

Look, there is no alternative to natural hygiene. Do not consider this as an alternative system of medicine on par with the prevalent system of medication to be resorted to when one is ill and to be given up when one is apparently well. In your own interest take to natural hygiene as a fish takes to water, understand the implications of natural hygiene to the fullest extent, adopt it in your daily life unmindful of the opinions of the people around. But adopt the total approach and not a fragmentary one.

Life power and vitality

The reputed saint, Sri Aurbindo Ghose once said: *"Living is experiencing the wholeness of our being; all else is existence."* How many of us are experiencing this blissful state? Are not most in the modern world only existing? What can we do to have this experience during the lifetime of ours? The science of natural hygiene can practically help us to achieve the purpose in view. This science tells us in no uncertain terms that life power or *prana shakti* functions in each living organism and is a gift of Mother Nature to every one of us. This power cannot be obtained from anywhere else in the world and is the most valuable possession as life depends upon it.

It is there in everyone of us as a vital reserve. A very small part of it is given to us every morning for carrying on that day's activities in the world. And this is vitality or *jeevan shakti*. The science of natural hygiene firmly asserts that economising the expenditure of vitality is the only means for maintaining health and for regaining health (in the case of those people who happen to be ill at present). In fact, our contention is that all medicaments (prescribed through various systems of medication ostensibly to cure patients) rob patients of their vitality and hence are totally unscientific.

If the modern man happens to suffer from chronic and destructive diseases, it is because his lifestyle is such as to lead to wastage of vitality in daily living. Logically getting back to normalcy in such cases would be possible only when the wasteful practices stop, giving place to near-ideal living. This is the reason why we insist on the practice of vital economy in daily life. This is why we appeal to patients to take to non-violent applications, as every violent application will lead to further enervation.

In practicing this vital economy we have to ensure the supply of the basic needs of living to the person in proper proportion.

The basic needs of living are:

- *Physical*: Constitution, activity (function, exercise, work), structural integrity of organs, functional efficiency of the different systems, cool air, water, food, sunshine, sleep (relaxation, repose, rest), posture, cleanliness.

- *Mental*: Integrity at mental level (clarity, character, positive attitude), activity (work), faith (in the fundamental goodness of Nature), proper attitude towards one's daily work, observance of orderliness and systematic discharge of work, happiness, etc.

A balanced supply of the basic needs of living is what is required to ensure normalcy of activity—this is what the term health implies. Where due to imperfect understanding a person lays stress upon just two or three factors (e.g. proper food, morning walk, exercise) and where consequently many other essential factors are not taken care of to the degree required, maintenance of/improvement in the health level cannot be experienced. And where some of the basic needs are not supplied to the extent required, even the observance of vital economy would not be practicable. Hence, we insist on sufficient care being exercised by an individual to ensure that all basic needs of living are supplied in a balanced manner.

In modern days, 'experts' in particular fields of knowledge tend to overemphasise, misleading the health-seeker by saying that their standpoint alone is important if one wants to be healthy. For instance, an 'expert' on yogasana and pranayama says that regular performance of certain yogasana *and* pranayama *are* sine-qua-non *of a healthy life. Another expert stresses upon 'meditation'. A third one says that food is all-important. The fourth one insists on just one point, like chewing of food.*

While what each one of the above is saying is correct so far as it goes, the human tendency to neglect the other essential points would complicate matters and lead to ill-health in due course of time.

Let no one belong to the category of the 'six blind men', where each insists that he alone is correct and the others are wrong, while the real fact is that no one had seen the whole elephant. Hence my plea is that every health-seeker should adopt the total approach on the subject of health maintenance/ health recovery. When such total approach is there, man would so order his daily life as to enable the establishment of orderliness within the organism.

Order and the Ordainer

Establishment of the order referred to above would set a

person on progressive improvement in his health level and where such an order becomes an established practice in one's day-to-day life, the principle of vital economy is observed to the last degree. No organ could in those circumstances be subjected to any violence. The science of natural hygiene has probed deeply into this subject and has set out clear guidelines to modern health-seekers on how to maintain this order within the system.

Everything in this world goes on in an orderly manner so long as man through his antics does not disturb the balance in Nature. The science of ecology recognises this fundamental truth and calls upon man not to indulge in his attempts to disturb this balance in Nature. The unpleasant features or disorders observed in the modern world are just man-made ones. Left to Nature, the order can be maintained all through in all aspects.

As the subject under discussion is man's health, the order that ought to be there should be the somatic awareness that ought to be present in every living cell of the human body, the symbiotic relationship among the different systems in the body and under the full control of life power or *prana shakti* which is the Ordainer within.

The rather unfortunate fact of man's suffering from chronic and destructive diseases is primarily due to the meaningless waste of life power within in various ways which are foisted on immature minds through what goes by the name of 'modern civilisation'.

Logic tells us that proper care exercised by man in redesigning his pattern of life can re-establish the order within and make him healthy.

Let the discerning individuals who can distinguish between the chaff and the grain spurn away the chaff by ensuring a balanced supply of the basic needs of living. Let the subject of natural hygiene be studied in depth, let the basic truth of this science be ever borne in mind and let life in this world be lived purposefully. This is the ardent wish of the writer.

The so-called holistic way

As lack of any positive result through the different systems of medication is experienced by more and more patients in the modern world, they switch over to Nature cure in the hope that the disease could be cured thus.

As these persons take to Nature cure only as an alternative system of medicine, there are a number of Nature-curists ready to oblige them. Though the system is getting more and more popular, its real significance and objective are forgotten, both by the practitioner and the patient. This is not a very desirable development but this is what is happening in the modern world. The practitioners are anxious to produce 'immediate results' and with this sole objective, so many procedures are being adopted. Maybe in these procedures, no chemicals or poisons are being employed and on this ground the practitioners insist that every new procedure should also form part of the Nature cure approach to give the system a holistic colour.

The so-called holistic procedures recently introduced by many practitioners into the system of Nature cure and against which I raise my voice of protest are:

- acupuncture
- accupressure
- electrotherapy
- magnetotherapy
- reflexotherapy
- chromotherapy

I do not approve of the so-called *yogic kriyas* like the *kunjal, neti* (*jal, sutra, ghrit* included), *vasti kriya* and the

hathyogic procedures, *pranayama* like *bhastrika, kapalbhati,* etc.

As one who has gone deeply into the subject of Nature cure and with more than half a century of experience I would make bold to say that every one of the above procedures violates the law of cause and effect, the principle of vital economy and the principle of non-violence, all of which have a great bearing on regaining health, retaining health and improving it progressively. Apart from the applications (therapies) listed above, many persons are said to be following palmistry, astrology, astronomy, etc. If we look into original works (really forming a part of our Vedic culture) on this subject, I have all admiration for the noble souls (saints and sages) who had done intense internal research and presented to humanity.

I should not, in the circumstances, object to the use of these sciences by the opportunists (lacking a dedicated knowledge on the subject) in adopting treatment that gives them immediate symptomatic relief. To the extent that these are being applied in a very cursory manner, the patients take these procedures also as remedies wherein the reverence to the original sciences is totally lost sight of. And here is the most objectionable aspect in applying these fragmentary procedures. Either give up the fragmentary approach or get authorities on these sciences adopt the total approach recommended by them. In short, any procedure adopted just as a remedy 'dealing with present problem/issue' can never be holistic.

The term holistic is being used very loosely and none is concerned about the following major issues involved in 'polluting' the science of Nature cure:

- Don't the perversions introduced into the system of Nature cure go against the fundamental philosophy of the science (which is to the effect that it is a way of life and not a system of treatment of diseases)?

- Don't these procedures inflict violence on any organ in the human body and as such are these not as bad as, if not worse than, drugs/chemicals advocated by the different medications?
- Don't everyone of these procedures occasion wastage—let everyone remember the truth that wastage is in every case anti-natural—of the vital power in the organism?
- Is not each of these procedures a remedy for giving immediate symptomatic relief and thus goes against the law of cause and effect, a fundamental natural law characteristic of the approach advocated by the science of Nature cure?
- As patients adopt one of these procedures which would only be remedy-minded, would they care to reform their diet or change their earlier habits of living the hygienic way?
- As no disease (whatever its nomenclature) can be radically cured without removing the basic cause thereof (viz. the enervating habits) and as these so-called holistic methods by occasioning immediate symptomatic relief to the patient make them, the patient forgets the real duty is to radically change his habit of living the hygienic way.
- Would not the application of these holistic procedures result in the loss of structural integrity of one or the other vital organs inside?
- Would not the application of these holistic procedures impair the functional efficiency of the different systems in the human organism?

To the practitioners and the patients alike I would like to pose a question: "In case your resorting to one or the other of the so-called holistic procedures is going to thwart the development of Nature cure as a science, would you like to be a party to this unprincipled and illogical development (though immediately no relief is being obtained by the patients this way)?"

I am sure you would not like to be a party to pervert the future of the Nature cure movement. Are you not aware of the effective methods to give immediate relief to the patients, keeping in view the need for radically healing the disease as quickly as possible?

I believe you all can have even immediate symptomatic relief without any of these holistic procedures and you will stand to fully benefit by adopting the basic Nature cure (which is but a synonym for natural hygiene).

The 'basic Nature cure' approach

Apart from what has already been expained earlier, all that is needed is the reader (let him be a practitioner or patient) should read in between the lines, meditate on the issues involved and come to the firm conclusion that the future generations should not accuse you of being a guilty party to have perverted this wonderful science.

Anyone wanting to benefit fully by following this basic Nature cure should avoid the one great error that they commit by mistaking the different applications in Nature cure as the only factors which could help in recovering from disease. Better keep away from the fragmentary approach and take only to the total approach.

Arise, awake, stop not till the goal is reached.